D0596713

100
PLUS

Also by Sonia Arrison

Telecrisis (editor)
Digital Dialogue

100
PLUS

HOW THE COMING AGE OF LONGEVITY WILL CHANGE EVERYTHING, FROM CAREERS AND RELATIONSHIPS TO FAMILY AND FAITH

SONIA ARRISON

BASIC BOOKS
A Member of the Perseus Books Group
New York

Published by Basic Books,
A Member of the Perseus Books Group

Books published by Basic Books are available at special discounts for bulk purchases in the United States by corporations, institutions, and other organizations. For more information, please contact the Special Markets Department at the Perseus Books Group, 2300 Chestnut Street, Suite 200, Philadelphia, PA 19103, or call (800) 810-4145, ext. 5000, or e-mail special.markets@perseusbooks.com.

Designed by Trish Wilkinson
Set in 11.5 point Goudy Old Style

Library of Congress Cataloging-in-Publication Data

Arrison, Sonia.
    100 plus : how the coming age of longevity will change everything : from careers and relationships to family and faith / Sonia Arrison.
        p.   cm.
    Includes bibliographical references and index.
    ISBN 978-0-465-01966-3 (hardcover : alk. paper)—
ISBN 978-0-465-02770-5 (ebook) 1. Longevity. 2. Life spans (Biology) 3. Social change. I. Title. II. Title: One hundred plus.
QP85.A77 2011
612.6'8—dc23   2011016674

10 9 8 7 6 5 4 3 2

To my grandparents, Mollie and Ralph, who inspired this book.
And to my husband, Aydin, and son, Henry,
for their continual love and support.

Contents

Foreword	*The Problem of Death* by Peter Thiel	*ix*
CHAPTER 1	Humankind's Eternal Quest for the Fountain of Youth	1
CHAPTER 2	How Science and Technology Will Increase Life Span	21
CHAPTER 3	Mother Nature and the Longevity Revolution	49
CHAPTER 4	The Longevity Divide: Does Living Longer Mean Living Better?	77
CHAPTER 5	The Changing Face of Family	101
CHAPTER 6	The Financial Implications of Longevity	127
CHAPTER 7	The Afterlife Versus a Longer Life: Religion in the Age of Longevity	151
CHAPTER 8	Leadership for a Longer-Lived World	175
Notes		*199*
Index		*237*

Foreword

The Problem of Death

OVER THE WHOLE history of our world, about 100 billion human beings have been born to see and experience the wonder of life. Only 7 billion remain alive today. The rest have perished. One hundred thousand more pass away every day; the most common causes, at least in the advanced countries, are diseases related to aging. In 2011 fewer than 1 in 10,000 people lived to see their hundredth birthday. Euphemistically, these terrible things are called the facts of life. It would be far more accurate to call them the problem of death.

With piercing clarity, I still recall the day I first learned of the problem of death. I was three years old. I was sitting on a rug in the living room of my parents' modest apartment in Cleveland, Ohio. I was at the age where I was asking my dad lots of questions.

"Where did the rug come from?"

"It came from a cow."

"What happened to the cow?"

"The cow died."

"What is death?"

"It means that the cow is no longer alive. Death happens to all animals. It also happens to all people. It will one day happen to me. It will one day happen to you."

My father seemed sad as he was saying these things. I remember that it was a very sad and disturbing day for me. I did not want my dad to die. And the world seemed too happy and wonderful a place to leave.

But human beings are not cows. For present purposes let me mention one key difference: unlike the other animals, we have knowledge of death. The origins of language, of culture, and of religion can perhaps all be traced to that point in the distant past when our ancestors first acquired this terrible knowledge and needed to tell themselves stories to make sense of life and death. Every myth on this planet is an untrue story that tells people that the purpose of life is death. Nationalist myths tell us that it is sweet and fitting to die for one's country, ideological myths tell us that progress requires violence and that one must break some eggs to make an omelet, and religious myths tell us to worship the old, the ancient, and the spirits of the dead.

The crisis of the modern world is the crisis of mythology. We no longer believe in the old stories about life and death, but we also cannot go back to a time when we were not yet human and did not know about death. We cannot go back in time and become two-year-olds, and we would prefer not to be turned into cows. At the same time, we cannot simply deal with death as a "fact of life." What we desperately need is a new story—a true story—to help make sense of the world in which we find ourselves.

————————

MY GOOD FRIEND Sonia Arrison offers a new story that makes more sense of the world by replacing solace with a challenge. From her perch as a technology analyst at the Pacific Research Institute in Silicon Valley, Arrison has been at the nexus of the future for the better part of two decades. Over the years the two of us have debated and discussed many of the cutting-edge questions in the technology world, but our conversations have always returned to the most important of questions: of how technology will change the balance between life and death.

Since the myths of the past and the present have been exposed, Arrison argues, we must follow the critical path forward: if we cannot forget or accept decline, then we must fight it and work to create a future no longer dominated by aging and death. The time has come for death to die.

Arrison began her work in public policy with a focus on computer technologies and the Internet, and it is perhaps worth highlighting the key difference between computer science and biological science, as traditionally understood: computers involve bits and reversible processes; biology involves stuff and seemingly irreversible processes. But computational power will soon be brought to bear on more and more domains, up to and including biological domains beginning with areas like genomics, protein folding, and modeling but culminating in a deeper understanding of life that will enable us to reverse all human ailments in the same way that we can fix the bugs of a computer program. Unlike the world of stuff, in the world of bits the arrow of time can be turned backward. Death will eventually be reduced from a mystery to a solvable problem. In this reduction we may hope that human life will achieve a new level of freedom and consciousness.

Arrison's book begins with a history of the many great men and women of the past who sought human longevity. She surveys the current generation of scientists and technologists who promise to usher in a new era, demonstrating that aging is a foe that can be hobbled and potentially even beaten. From here Arrison goes to the heart of things by directly confronting opposition to longer and healthier lives and outlining the extraordinary economic, social, and cultural changes that will happen as the world wakes up from history. Although Arrison considers a world where individuals will have their life expectancies extended to 150 years, the logic of her work leads to the more speculative question of the final conquest of death.

We may wonder whether triumph over death may also mean the end of science in the twofold sense of "end" as both culmination and termination. It will be a culmination because the end of aging and death would mean the final mastery of science over nature or chance. And it would also perhaps represent a termination because the greatest driver for scientific progress in the modern world will be no more. In the end, the Tree of Life may prove more desirable than the Tree of Knowledge, but for now we must begin with the latter to find our way back to the former.

———

QUESTIONS OF LIFE and death have vexed humanity for millennia. There is a tendency to respond to these questions with opposite (but strangely related) extremes of despair or complacency: we may despair of solving the problem of aging and give up, or we may become complacent about the problem of aging and so not try. To my mind, the most important aspect of the book involves the way in which Arrison's approach to the problem—her incredible style, if you will—charts the substantive path forward to avoid these twin shoals. Let me end with a few thoughts on how to avoid each.

The most insidious form of despair makes a claim about nature—that aging and death are somehow natural or that "all that lives must die," as Hamlet's evil mother, Gertrude, rationalizes away the rottenness that is Denmark. Arrison dispatches this claim by reminding us that the very question of nature must be asked in earnest and answered with action. Properly, few things are less natural than *not* to rage against the dying of the light. The struggle against aging is therefore the most natural thing we could possibly do. It is the most humane, and the most human, of struggles. Arrison fights despair by urging us to become more like ourselves, to become more human than we already are.

The most insidious form of complacency makes a claim about other people—that aging and death will be solved by others and that we are mere spectators to the unfolding of technology. But the future is not determined. We cannot (or should not) outsource our own lives. In whatever capacity we can—as intellectuals, scientists, investors, voters, cultural leaders—we must take ownership of the future. In order to win, we must fight. We are not mere spectators, and Arrison is no mere prophet. Instead, she truly is a great general, who is marshaling all of the vast forces of humanity in its titanic struggle against the Great Enemy of the world, whose true name is Death. I look forward to the battle being joined.

Death was natural in the past, but so was the instinct to fight it. The future only has room for one of them.

Peter Thiel
Spring 2011
San Francisco

CHAPTER 1

Humankind's Eternal Quest for the Fountain of Youth

DR. TYRELL: What seems to be the problem?
ROY: Death.

—*Blade Runner*

FOR AS LONG as humans have been around, they have dreamed about living forever. Now, for the first time in history, science is bringing humanity closer to realizing that dream through advances that could potentially add hundreds of years to the average life span. This pivotal moment in time is not the random result of chance. Instead, it follows directly from a vast culture of human imagination and action directed toward the proverbial fountain of youth.

Pop culture fans will remember how androids in the classic movie *Blade Runner* created havoc over their limited life spans—unlike humans, they had not devised creative ways of dealing with the unpleasant issue of death. Religion has long been a buffer for this anxiety-filled topic, and when looking at the subject through the lens of human imagination and creativity, there are three typical responses. Some people convince themselves to accept death because it is humanity's punishment for not living pious or healthy lives. Others embrace death because they believe it would be dangerous to do otherwise. And then there are those who actively attempt to overcome it. Given that vanquishing death has been a fascination for centuries, it would be impossible to cover everything relating to this topic, so instead this book will examine some of the most famous stories, myths, and actual experiments aimed at living longer. This will set the stage for a larger discussion about how long science will extend our lives and how that in turn will change our ecological, social, financial, and religious worlds.

IT'S OUR FAULT

According to the Bible, Adam and Eve made a huge mistake that affected the future of all humans coming after them: they disobeyed God and ate the forbidden fruit of the Tree of Knowledge of good and evil. This made God so angry that He kicked them out of the Garden of Eden, where they would have been immortal, and thrust them into a world where sickness, starvation, and other ills could befall them and their kin. Death was the price of surrender to temptation. In following the logic of this story, many have concluded that Adam and Eve are to blame for our relatively short eighty-year life expectancy, but surprisingly, even after their mistake, humans lived a long time according to the Bible.

The oldest person the Bible mentions is Methuselah, who lived 969 years, but there were others whose life spans were also exceptional. Methuselah's grandson Noah, who built the ark, lived 950 years. Adam reached 930, and his son Seth and grandson Enos lived to 912 and 905, respectively. These sky-high numbers must have been a source of disappointment for Moses, who, the Bible notes, lived to be only 120 years, a shorter length of time than the oldest modern (and verified) person, Jeanne Calment of France, who died at 122 in 1997.[1] So how do Judeo-Christian believers explain the big discrepancy in life span between Adam's time and now?

Thirteenth-century English philosopher Roger Bacon, often referred to as the father of longevity science, thought he had an answer. He believed that humanity's shorter life span was due to immoral behavior and bad habits.[2] Although he was a friar, he advocated open science and believed that life span could be extended, writing a treatise titled "The Cure of Old Age, and Preservation of Youth."[3] According to historian Lucian Boia, Bacon advocated an Atkin's-like diet "based on meat, egg yolks, and red wine."[4] And even though shorter life spans were mostly humanity's fault, Bacon also thought that as the earth got older, it didn't provide as well for the humans on it, thus resulting in shorter life spans.[5]

Alcohol consumption was considered to be another cause for humans' untimely demise, but this theory was as hotly contested back then as it is now. Medical historian David Boyd Haycock points out that "alcohol was often blamed for shortening human life spans. The Bible makes it clear that, following the Flood, Noah was the first person ever to cultivate grapes and make wine. It did not take a genius to note that it was also since the age of Noah that life spans had begun their sudden decline."[6] On the opposite side of this issue were people like Tobias Whitaker, one of King Charles II's physicians, who wrote a book about how wine could be used to lengthen life span.[7] The argument between these two points of view is still with us: some science shows that alcohol use causes cancer, and other studies focus on the "French paradox," in which wine is thought to protect eaters of high-fat French food from heart disease. Although the focus thus far has been on biblical sources, stories involving other gods and faiths similarly stressed the idea that disobedience, bad habits, and immoral behavior shortened life span.

For instance, in Greek mythology, humans are to blame through their association with a mischievous and disobedient god, Prometheus. Known as a trickster, Prometheus decides to give the ruling god, Zeus, an ox that is all fat and bones but no meat. Understandably, this angers Zeus, and in retaliation he decides to take fire away from humans because Prometheus is known to be fond of them. In response, Prometheus steals fire and brings it back to humans, but this only angers Zeus more, leading him to create the first woman, named Pandora, who is beautiful and charming but carries a lethal jar. As most people know, the story ends with Zeus giving Pandora to humans, after which she opens her jar, unleashing disease, suffering, and death.[8] If humans had only associated with better-behaved gods, life might be longer.

Piety and obedience also surface in Taoist thought as key to longevity. Early Taoists believed that life could be lengthened if people adhered to certain rules. Historian Gerald Gruman notes that for dedicated Taoists looking to extend life, "not only were grains prohibited but also meat, wine, and many vegetables." But the real drama, he says, came from the concept of the "Three Worms" living inside each person and "hinder[ing] the perfectibility of man," much like Adam and Eve's original sin.[9] He writes that "the Three Worms were pictured as keeping a careful account of misdeeds, which they regularly reported to heaven to persuade the gods to decrease the life span of the host."[10] Not only a person's actions but also her willpower has been thought to have a direct impact on life span. Italian priest St. Thomas Aquinas believed that willpower was the key to longevity. After all, it was lack of willpower that had gotten Adam and Eve into the perilous position of eating from the tree of knowledge in the first place, so maybe willpower was the cure for their descendants. "The implication," argue S. Jay Olshansky and Bruce A. Carnes in their book *The Quest for Immortality*, "is that by reasserting control over the mind, the supernatural power taken by God could be restored."[11] This idea of mind over matter was, and still is, shared by many as powerful medicine and certainly isn't limited to the religious sphere. The very fact of a placebo effect, in which people's symptoms subside simply because they think they are taking a drug when they are instead taking a sugar pill (the placebo), is a reminder of how powerful the mind can be. Such power led Irish writer George Bernard Shaw to advocate for the Lamarckian idea that characteristics could be acquired and passed down through generations. Hence, a giraffe's neck evolved over time, he reasoned, as members of each generation reached up, willing themselves to get the leaves on higher and higher branches. "The long necks," he explained, "were evolved by wanting and trying."[12] Apparently, Shaw thought that humans didn't try hard enough for long lives. He himself was a vegetarian and wound up living to age ninety-four, so by his own theory he may have "willed" a longer life.

Another tale about how the outcome of mortality can be traced back to the failure of human will is *The Epic of Gilgamesh*, which is one of the oldest known stories from Babylonia.[13] Gilgamesh is a king who is mean to his subjects, so the gods send him a distraction in the form of a warrior named Enkidu. After the two battle it out for a while, they earn each other's respect and become friends, but then Enkidu is sentenced to die after the two insult the gods. This causes Gilgamesh to become obsessed with avoiding death, and he goes on a journey to find a way to become immortal. He finds a sage named Utanapishtim, who tells him that there are two ways to cheat death. First, he can master sleep. If he can manage to stay awake for six days and seven nights, he will become immortal. But Gilgamesh is exhausted and falls asleep. There is one last chance for him to earn his immortality. He is told to swim to the bottom of the sea, find a box-thorn plant, and eat it. Gilgamesh does successfully find the plant and brings it to the surface, but before he eats it, he decides to rest and have a cool bath. This pit stop is costly because while he's bathing, a snake appears and gobbles up the plant, a literary explanation for why snakes have the regenerative power to shed their skin.

Willpower also has another role to play when it comes to sexual impulses and life span. Franco-American physiologist Charles-Edouard Brown-Séquard argued in 1889 that sex took years off people's lives. It was a "well known fact," he argued, "that seminal losses arising from any cause, produce a mental and physical debility which is in proportion to their frequency."[14] As with the controversy over wine's effect on life span, the effect of sex is debatable. Brown-Sequard's position was in direct opposition to the Taoist perspective, which said that "man does not want to be without woman; if he is without woman, he becomes agitated; if he becomes agitated, his spirits become fatigued; if his spirits become fatigued, his longevity is decreased."[15] The linkage of sex and death (in either a positive or a negative way) is common throughout the literature on longevity and has produced some rather strange proposed "treatments," as we will see when we start looking at the huge body of human action aimed at fighting death.

OVERCOMING DEATH, IMAGINING TRAGIC RESULTS

Even if we could devise a way to live longer, there are heaps of stories explaining why we wouldn't want to. Most of these stories focus on unintended consequences that end in tragedy. From a psychological perspective, such a storyline is not surprising because we humans are extremely good at rationalizing away things we can't control. That is, if we can convince ourselves that we wouldn't want to live longer, then it isn't so bad that we can't. In this vein, one of the best story-tellers of all time was Oscar Wilde.

Wilde's novel *The Picture of Dorian Gray* makes use of the element of the fantastic to present a morality tale about the unintended consequences of extended life. First serialized in 1890, *The Picture of Dorian Gray* was published in a full, revised edition in 1891. In the story, a young man named Dorian sits for a portrait by the artist Basil Hallward. During a conversation with a friend of Hallward's, Dorian comes to the realization that beauty is fleeting and that his own beauty and youth will inevitably fade. Rather than reconciling himself to this fact, Dorian wishes aloud that his portrait would age instead of him. His wish is magically granted, and he begins his soon-to-be-tragic life. The catch is that the portrait not only ages but also becomes more disfigured with every act of depravity Dorian commits.[16]

And commit acts of depravity he does. Freed from the physical consequences of his actions, Dorian begins a new life as a hedonist, seeking only pleasure. Dorian is not freed from the moral or emotional consequences of such a life, however, and he becomes increasingly bitter over his fate, eventually killing the artist Hallward in an act of vengeance-induced rage.[17] Dorian attempts to reform and tread a new path but finds that the aging and disfigurement of the portrait have only grown worse. Finally, he destroys the painting and instantly dies himself. His servants find his body aged to the point of being unidentifiable, while the painting portrays Dorian as he had been at the time of its creation. Wilde's story offers a theme common in popular literature: that extended life carries with it severe moral and ethical implications. Extending life span, he suggested, was not merely a physical act. It was also a moral one because if freed from the process of aging, a person would be largely freed from the physical consequences of his actions.[18] In Wilde's mind, immortality was a curse.

A related story is that of the sad Dr. Faust, whose passion for youth lands him in hell for all eternity. There have been many iterations of the Faust theme by various writers, but the first version appeared in 1587 by an anonymous German author. The general story is that Dr. Faust makes a bargain with the devil: in exchange for wealth and power, Faust sells his soul to the devil. Although the story dates back to 1587, it wasn't until Johann Wolfgang von Goethe took the legend up around 1770 that Dr. Faust joined the longevity literature. In Goethe's version, Faust seeks *youth* in addition to money and power. According to historian Lucian Boia, "Here Faust swallows a witch's potion designed to restore his youth and make him fall in love."[19] Goethe's play was followed by a popular 1859 opera by Charles Gounod that shows the "miracle of rejuvenation" on stage, after which the newly young man falls in love.[20]

Risking eternity in hell for youth is a bad decision, but other stories warn that extended longevity could turn people into monsters, potentially creating hell on earth. Vampires are perhaps *the* classic immortal monster. They live a long time, but the nasty side effect is that they become worse than animals, drinking blood and stealing the life essence of others to stay undead. Bram Stoker is famous for his Dracula stories along these lines and is credited with coining the term "undead."[21] Throughout history, vampires were mostly thought of as scary, shadowy creatures, but as anyone who pays attention to mass media knows, vampires are currently in vogue. Both the *Twilight* movie series and the HBO *True Blood* series have romanticized vampires, making them seem glamorous, powerful, and sexy. "The vampire is the new James Dean," Hollywood writer and executive producer Julie Plec told the *New York Times* in 2009.[22] But as *National Geographic* historian Mark Collins Jenkins points out, the idea of vampires stealing people's blood to maintain their existence has dark roots connected to real stories of disease and murder.

One of the more interesting stories is about a Slovakian countess named Elizabeth Bathory. According to the legend, when a drop of blood accidentally fell on her hand after she hit a servant, her skin magically looked younger. In an effort to create this effect on her entire body, the forty-year-old widow began a decade of butchery.[23] Although it's not plausible that the woman actually looked younger after getting blood on her hand, it is possible that she *thought* she looked younger and carried out a murder spree based on this belief. Indeed, Jenkins notes that historical records show that the king of Hungary presided over a real trial for the countess, and she was found guilty of eighty counts of murder.[24]

But vampires are not the only monsters associated with myths of longevity. There is also the story of Frankenstein. Children all over the world grow up with a cartoon version of a mad scientist creating a monster in his lab, but even though today's versions might be cute or even funny, Mary Shelley's 1818 original was not. In that story a scientist named Victor Frankenstein decides to create life out of pieces of dead body parts, which he infuses with the "spark of being."[25] The creature born from these parts is very ugly, and it wants to be accepted but isn't, so it becomes dangerous. It threatens its creator, Dr. Frankenstein, when he refuses to create another monster as a mate. "Beware, for I am fearless and therefore powerful. I will watch with the wiliness of a snake, that I may sting with its venom."[26] Clearly, this tale is a warning that attempting to reassemble life is going beyond where humans are meant to go. As biomedical humanities scholar Carol C. Donley notes, "In bringing life to dead body parts, Frankenstein crosses the border of natural limits, creating life or extending it far beyond its normal span."[27]

And if children aren't wary about longevity after reading *Frankenstein*, another classic now aimed at kids, *Gulliver's Travels*, makes the point loud and clear. In Jonathan Swift's satire, Gulliver visits the nation of Luggnagg, where a very small group of the inhabitants are born immortal. These "struldbrugs" can be identified by "a red circular spot in the forehead, directly over the left eyebrow."[28] Gulliver gets very excited by the prospect of people, even though rare, who can live forever. He gushes over the wisdom they must impart to the community and imagines what his life would be like if he were one of them.

"I cried out, as in a rapture," Gulliver exclaims. "Happy nation, where every child hath at least a chance for being immortal! Happy people, who enjoy so many living examples of ancient virtue, and have masters ready to instruct them in the wisdom of all former ages! but happiest, beyond all comparison, are those excellent *struldbrugs*, who, being born exempt from that universal calamity of human nature, have their minds free and disengaged, without the weight and depression of spirits caused by the continual apprehensions of death!"[29]

Alas, Gulliver has jumped to conclusions too fast. He is informed that being a struldbrug is actually a curse and that these immortals have a negative effect on society because they are not exempt from aging or disease. They "acted like mortals till about thirty years old; after which, by degrees, they grew melancholy and dejected, increasing in both till they came to fourscore." By eighty years old, they turn into nasty people and are "not only opinionative, peevish, covetous, morose, vain, talkative, but incapable of friendship, and dead to all natural affection, which never descended below their grandchildren." At ninety, they lose their teeth and hair, and because the language of the country continually evolves, the older struldbrugs can't "hold any conversation (farther than by a few general words) with their neighbours the mortals; and thus they lie under the disadvantage of living like foreigners in their own country."[30]

Swift's cutting satire of those who long to live forever was written at an inauspicious moment in time. As historian Haycock points out, life expectancy at birth was plummeting in England. In 1581, life expectancy was 42.7 years, but by the time that *Travels into Several Remote Nations of the World, by Lemuel Gulliver* was published in 1726, life expectancy was a depressing 25.3 years.[31] No wonder Swift had little patience for people who dreamed of immortality—things in his world were going in the wrong direction.

But Swift wasn't the only author to paint a horrid picture of living forever while growing old. It was the theme of many other cautionary tales, such as the ancient Greek story of Eos and Tithonus. Eos, the god of dawn, falls in love with a mortal man named Tithonus, who is a member of the Trojan royal house.[32] She asks Zeus to grant her lover immortality, and Zeus agrees. The two lovers are happy for years until it becomes apparent that Tithonus is aging. Unfortunately, Eos forgot to ask for agelessness, so Tithonus suffers at the hands of time, getting so weak and old that "there was nothing for Eos to do but shut him away in a room where he yet lies, babbling endlessly."[33] Becoming old and incompetent is not a fate anyone wishes for, and the role of a young immortal living among mortals is also a classic literary technique for arguing that humans shouldn't chase the dream of living forever.

Isaac Asimov told a story along these lines in his novella *The Bicentennial Man*, made into a movie starring Robin Williams in 1999. *The Bicentennial Man* is the story of an NDR-series robot named Andrew who is originally purchased by the Martin family to do chores. Clunky and socially awkward at first, Andrew eventually develops human-like abilities such as creativity and self-awareness. He bonds with the family, and as time goes on, he is upgraded, but each human generation dies, and he finds himself lonely, wishing he were human. Through his creativity, Andrew generates wealth, gains his freedom, and develops human prosthetic components to replace his mechanical ones so that he'll be more like the humans he lives among. He falls in love with the granddaughter of the daughter of his original family and wants to marry her, but they cannot be married because he is not recognized as a human. Eventually, when he has replaced enough of his body that he ages and dies like a human, the world congress validates his marriage and recognizes him as "the oldest living human in recorded history" at two hundred years old.[34]

But not all stories about the topic of longevity are so negative. Director Ron Howard's 1985 film *Cocoon* offered a new twist on the fountain of youth story and was a box office hit, winning two Academy Awards (for visual effects and acting).[35] *Cocoon* is the story of a group of retirement home residents who break into a nearby mansion to go swimming in its elaborate pool. After swimming, they discover that they are getting physically younger. Unbeknownst to them, the house has been rented by a group of aliens who have returned to earth after 10,000 years to retrieve comrades who were left behind during an earlier mission and have been preserved in podlike cocoons, living in a sort of suspended animation. The water in the pool is filled with an unspecified "life-force" that will rejuvenate the aliens and allow them to return home. The aliens discover the elderly swimmers but let them keep visiting as long as they promise not to disturb the cocoons in the water. They agree, but eventually word gets out and the pool is overflowing with people desperate to become younger again. Unfortunately, this many people in the pool kill the cocooned aliens. The remaining aliens decide to leave but offer to take the original group of retirement home residents with them; they will still feel young, they are told, and will never age. When asked if they'll live forever, the alien leader replies, "We don't know what forever is." The outcome in this case appears to be good for the residents who choose immortality, as the alien leader promises them that "the new civilizations you would be traveling to would be unlike anything you've ever seen before. But I promise you, you will all lead productive lives."[36] Here, rejuvenation is portrayed as an adventure and the opening of new possibilities rather than a punishment from which to be released. *This* is the longevity that humans have historically longed for, and it has fueled many types of actual attempts at extending human life. To these we will now turn.

FIGHTING DEATH

The old adage that actions speak louder than words provides an important bit of wisdom when it comes to analyzing the longevity landscape. For all the stories that humans have concocted to convince themselves that living longer isn't worthwhile, there are just as many stories about how humans have *actually* reached for the fountain of youth. Death is a problem for all of us, and whereas some accept it in various ways, others look for solutions.

Water has always been thought to be important to human longevity, resulting in myths of fountains of youth that could restore health, and real people have looked long and hard to find these eternal springs. Perhaps most famous of the fountain-chasers was Juan Ponce de León, a Spanish explorer who accidentally discovered Florida on his quest to find the springs of Bimini, which were rumored to have youth-extending properties. During his quest, members of the Council of the Indies who communicated often with Spanish explorers and officials believed and supported the theory that remedies to human illness and aging could be found in nature. Historian Gerald Gruman notes that an influential member of the Council of the Indies reasoned that "if Mother Nature provides means of rejuvenation to dumb animals like the snake, the eagle, and the crow, why should she not also create similar bounties for man."[37] A form of this thinking is alive and well today among serious researchers examining the biological mechanisms for how some animals, like salamanders, can regenerate parts of their bodies.[38]

Alexander the Great, who conquered a huge part of the world before he died in 323 BC, was also rumored to have been looking for a fountain of youth. Many myths based on his life were generated, one of the most interesting of which said that Alexander's cook accidentally discovered the fountain when a dead fish he was going to prepare suddenly became alive again. The cook immediately jumped in the water and became immortal. When Alexander asked for the location of the spring, the cook wouldn't reveal it, so Alexander tossed him into the sea, where he lived on in demonic form.[39] Of course, Alexander's failure to discover a fountain of youth hasn't discouraged countless numbers of people from searching land and sea for life-extending compounds.

To this day, naturalists, scientists, and yes, quacks, have looked for and promoted various ways that nature can help to extend life. Aside from water, various salts, muds, herbs, and even metals have been touted for their detoxifying and healing properties. This leads us to a discussion about alchemists. Known to most people today as the tricksters who attempted to make silver and gold out of other metals, alchemists were obsessed with longevity and were found concocting elixirs all over the world, including China, India, the Near East, England, France, and Denmark. But they weren't thought of as hucksters; instead, they were well regarded in their communities. As Olshansky and Carnes note, top alchemists hobnobbed with the elite, were paid extremely well for their elixirs, and generally led upscale lives.[40] They heated the red powder of cinnabar, and it became a sought-after silvery mercury. They also thought that ingesting gold and other metals such as mercury could lengthen one's life. We now know that mercury is extremely toxic, but back then the liquid metal seemed magical.

Qin Shi Huang, the first emperor of China, was convinced that mercury could lengthen his life, and England's Henry VI gave special permission to three men to create a medicine that would be so amazing that "all curable infirmities would be easily cured by it."[41] How long could a person who followed the advice of the alchemists live? The famous alchemist Paracelsus argued against a set limit, "so long as the right medicine . . . could be found to cure disease and maintain health."[42] Gold, mercury, herbs, tobacco, and opiates were all possible medicines in this quest. Snakes were also an ingredient in some elixirs, either the water that they swam in or a concoction made from them. They were thought to possess strong rejuvenation properties because of their ability to shed their skin.[43] Such powers led respected thinkers to recommend medicines made from snakes, but sometimes such attempts at extending life went badly wrong. In 1633, the wife of a well-regarded Royal Society fellow died from drinking "viper wine," and she was not the only one to have suffered in a life-extension experiment.[44]

Philosopher and author Francis Bacon (no relation to Roger) became deeply interested in life extension. Like Aristotle before him, Bacon thought that aging was due to a shifting in a spiritlike essence in the body, but he deviated from the Greek philosopher's path by thinking that the human body could be repaired.[45] Bacon theorized that to extend life, the human spirit or flame could not escape the body but had to be kept cool enough so that the heat from this flame didn't damage the person from inside. Therefore, he reasoned, to keep one's life force, a person needed to take cold baths and use oil to close the pores.[46] At the same time, a person should cool the flame with drugs like opium and tobacco.[47] Ironically, Bacon eventually died chasing the longevity-related idea that cool temperatures would preserve flesh the same way they preserved such things as fruit. In 1626, at the age of sixty-five, when he was already frail and unhealthy, he suddenly asked his driver to stop on the side of the road in the cold of winter to buy a chicken. The two of them had the chicken killed and cleaned, and Bacon frantically stuffed the bird with snow in an effort to test his hypothesis. He immediately came down with chills and other nasty symptoms, landing him in his deathbed.[48] But just because Bacon wound up dying following his hunches doesn't mean he lacked some good ideas. As we know, cold does indeed preserve flesh, which is why we all now use refrigerators, especially for meat. Bacon also theorized about organ transplants and blood transfusions, two ideas that would have been quite shocking at the time but are now common procedures.[49]

Not long after Bacon suggested blood transfusions, one was actually attempted. In 1650, physician Richard Lower conducted the first successful blood transfusion on dogs.[50] It didn't take much imagination for those looking for new rejuvenation techniques to come to the conclusion that "young" blood might help reinvigorate the old. According to Royal Society papers, an old dog given blood from a young spaniel was "perfectly cured."[51] Then, in 1667, the first transfusion to a human (using lamb's blood) was performed by Jean Denis, but his work stopped following the death of one of his patients. The technique was not really put into use until the nineteenth century.[52] We now know that animal blood is not a possible substitute for human blood, and even good ideas like blood transfusions, which today have saved millions of lives, can be put on hold for long periods if experiments based on them aren't conducted properly and are viewed as strange and dangerous.

A less messy way to try achieving longer life came in the form of astrology and matching "one's life to the movements of the stars."[53] A seventeenth-century astrologer at the court of the elector of Brandenburg told his patrons that changing location and diet based on the stars would help them avoid harm.[54] Some people today still believe that they can live longer and better lives by reading their horoscopes, even though the "wisdom" that astrologers offer is relegated to the entertainment section of the newspaper.

The practice of yoga has also been purported to increase longevity, and there are tales of yogis living for well over a hundred years. Scholar Mircea Eliade, one of the foremost interpreters of yoga to Western audiences, argues that, even though immortality was not originally a concern of yogic practice, it later became connected. At some point, he argues, yoga was identified with magic and in particular "with the magical means of vanquishing death."[55] Horoscopes and yoga might be associated in different ways with magic, but for those people not impressed with these options, the more earthly idea of changing diet is another nonmessy practice that many have tried.

As we have already seen, thinkers like Roger Bacon had ideas about the proper diet for longevity, and he was certainly not alone in thinking that what humans put in their bodies influences the length of their life. Another prominent scientist obsessed with diet was Elie

Metchnikoff, who won a Nobel Prize for his work in immunology. He thought that the way to a long life could be found through ingesting sour milk or Bulgarian yogurt because it contains lactic acid, which kills harmful microbes in our bodies.[56] Humans' long intestine is a problem, he reasoned, because it is loaded with bacteria and waste. In a 1908 article, the *New York Times* wrote about Metchnikoff's ideas with great enthusiasm, saying, "Elie Metchnikoff declares human existence may be indefinitely extended—There are realms of life in which death is not natural."[57]

Yogurt may not be a miracle drug, but it is a commonly accepted notion that what people eat affects their health. Today, there are tons of books on the market that purport to have the answer to eating for a long life, such as *The Longevity Diet*, *The Okinawa Diet Plan*, *The Blue Zones*, *Beyond the 120 Year Diet*, *The Advanced Mediterranean Diet*, and *The CR Way*. Although most diets cannot prove they actually help to fight aging, there is some evidence to suggest that caloric restriction can have an impact on life expectancy, the science of which we will explore in the next chapter. For now, it will suffice to say that caloric restriction is exactly what it sounds like— eating a lot less food.

Even though restricting diet is a difficult proposition for many, perhaps a worse fate was suffered by those who agreed to receive grafts of chimpanzee testicles. In 1920, Serge Voronoff, a Russian doctor based in Paris, started transplanting parts of chimps in an effort to restore youth to men under the theory that the sex glands drove energy.[58] We have seen that the linking of sex and youth is not a new idea, but the use of animal transplants in this way was fairly novel. Many of Dr. Voronoff's patients died, but those who didn't thought they actually saw results (most likely a placebo effect). And he wasn't the only one wedded to this theory. In America, doctors in prisons were experimenting with similar techniques. Eventually, some well-known people underwent similar procedures, including former middleweight champion boxer Frank Klaus and Irish poet William Butler Yeats.[59] Indeed, Yeats felt the placebo effect so strongly that the sixty-nine-year-old entered into an affair with a twenty-seven-year-old actress.[60]

We now know that grafting animal tissue onto humans is useless because the body rejects it, but we have also learned a lot more about the endocrine system and the impact that hormones have on our bodies. How exactly hormones affect aging is still up in the air, but judging from the rise in the market for human growth hormone (HGH) and bioidentical hormone replacement therapy, we can clearly see that there is a very large group of people who are not content to sit around and wait for studies to be conducted. Like Klaus and Yeats, these individuals see that their time is limited, and when they begin to sense the end closing in, they are willing to take risks, even though government organizations like the Food and Drug Administration have banned the use of HGH for antiaging purposes. Actor Sylvester Stallone is a Hollywood example of someone who got into trouble for taking HGH when authorities in Australia confiscated his supply and fined him $10,651.[61] Yet even after the debacle, he defended his decision to take the hormone, saying, "The most important thing about HGH—and I think more people should be aware of this—is it really takes off the wear and tear that your body takes. The power to recuperate is very, very limited. So all it does is expedite."[62] Actress Suzanne Somers is another modern believer in hormone therapy, so much so that she wrote a book titled *Ageless: The Naked Truth About Bioidentical Hormones*. She argues that hormone therapy is not like "practicing voodoo, it's not hippie treatment, it's not granola—it's cutting-edge. . . . It's the key to the fountain of youth for internal health and external beauty."[63] To what extent hormones affect aging will be revealed over the years, but the point is that humans have long been and still are actively attempting to figure out how to stay younger and healthier for longer, and hormones are one of the areas still actively gaining proponents for experimentation, despite detractors.

Another, even more controversial, method of attempting to extend life span was imagined by inventor Benjamin Franklin in a letter he wrote to his friend Dr. Jacques Barbeu-Dubourg in 1773: "I

wish it were possible, from this instance, to invent a method of em-
balming drowned persons, in such a manner that they may be recalled to life at any period, however distant; for having a very ardent
desire to see and observe the state of America a hundred years hence,
I should prefer to any ordinary death the being immersed in a cask of
Madeira wine, with a few friends, till that time, to be then recalled to
life by the solar warmth of my dear country."[64]

Franklin was essentially forecasting the idea of suspended animation, now known as cryonics, in which humans are frozen in the
hope that they can later be revived when science has advanced far
enough to "reanimate" someone and cure his terminal disease. This
might sound more like science fiction than reality, particularly
because the idea was inspired by Neil Ronald Jones's 1931 story
"The Jameson Satellite," in which a professor was sent into outer
space and then brought back to life by aliens.[65] But fiction is where
ideas often start, and Jones's story inspired scientifically minded
thinkers such as Robert Ettinger, who penned *The Prospect of Immortality*, which promoted the idea of freezing people. The cover of
Ettinger's book boldly told readers that the "Prospect of Immortality
is a sober, scientific, and logical argument founded on undeniable
fact: that a body deep-frozen stands a better chance of being revived
than one rotting in the ground; and that many people who died fifty
or a hundred years ago of 'incurable' diseases would today be
cured."[66] The science behind cryonics has actually become better
over time, and there is now a process called vitrification that converts liquids into a glasslike state (glass doesn't expand like ice
does), as opposed to earlier methods that damaged tissues and cells
because ice was the result of simple freezing. In September 2009,
U.S. scientists published a paper detailing how they had frozen a
rabbit kidney using vitrification and then successfully thawed and
transplanted the organ.[67] If the process can be refined so that it
doesn't poison human organs with the chemicals being used, it
could be possible to store human organs for transplants that otherwise might have been wasted because the donor was in a different

location from the recipient. Of course, the science of full-body cry-onics is a long way off, but the point here, as in all of the previous examples and stories, is that humanity's strong imagination is the engine of innovation driving the science that will extend our lives.

Living longer in a healthy state has been the collective dream of humanity for ages. The concept of death produces great anxiety, which has helped to inspire creative thinkers and motivate real action. One way to resolve this anxiety is to accept our fate under the reasoning that somehow humans are responsible for it. Whether humans angered a god or just didn't follow proper dietary and other rules, death is our fault. Another way to tackle the issue is to imagine that nasty things would happen if we were to extend our lives, and many characters, like vampires, Frankenstein's monster, and Jonathan Swift's struldbrugs, are examples of these horrible results. A third method is to attack the issue head-on and attempt various experiments to make humans longer-lived and healthy. As we have seen in this chapter, many such experiments are failures, but each failure is a lesson, and humanity is now much closer to walking down the right path. It is to current scientific ideas, no doubt informed by the huge literature already discussed, that we will now turn.

CHAPTER 2

How Science and Technology
Will Increase Life Span

ONE OF HUMANITY'S greatest achievements is the extension of the average life span.[1] Consider that for a person born during the Cro-Magnon era, life expectancy was a meager eighteen years.[2] By the time of the European Renaissance, a person could expect to see thirty birthdays, and by 1850 that number had risen to forty-three.[3] Now, people born in Western societies can expect close to eighty birthdays and look forward to more as science and technology advance (see Figure 2.1). Humanity persists in chasing longer life and greater health, and even though the gains so far have been significant, even more dramatic possibilities await.

We are at the cusp of a revolution in medicine and biotechnology that will radically increase not just our life spans but also, and more importantly, our *health* spans. That is, we will live longer and with a higher quality of life. This chapter will examine the fascinating new technologies that will allow doctors to repair or replace worn-out body parts, re-engineer our bodies, and take preventative measures that will radically lengthen our lives. The concept that human bodies are like machines is certainly not new; what has changed is that new tools with better instructions have been discovered.

21

FIGURE 2.1

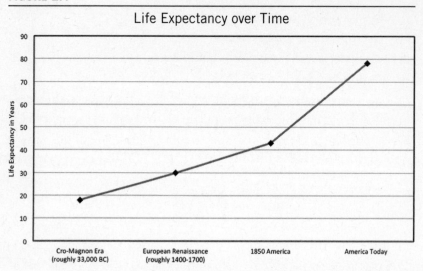

Life Expectancy over Time

REDEFINING OLD AGE

Before discussing how new technologies will allow us to live longer, it makes sense for readers to briefly examine how life expectancies have been extended thus far. Tragically, the majority of children used to die before reaching adulthood.[4] This was mainly due to infectious diseases, poor nutrition, and sanitation problems. Discoveries such as antibiotics, vaccines, vitamins, and indoor plumbing led to humanity's rapid gains in life expectancy. What this means is that for most of history gains in human life expectancy were made at the beginning, not the end, of life. It is true that older people have always been part of society, but they were less numerous and more weathered than today's seniors. As life expectancy rose, so did the number of older people, and that was when chronic diseases associated with aging, such as heart disease, cancer, and Alzheimer's, made their way into our common life and vocabulary. But that is not the end of the story. Rather, it is the beginning of a new chapter in which humanity takes on ill health and death at later ages. Already, there is good news on this front.

Some scholars used to think that extending life at younger ages was inevitable but that making progress at older ages wasn't possible. Curing infectious diseases was one thing, but taking on heart disease, cancer, and, ultimately, aging was quite another, the thinking went. The idea of a "natural," set life span clouded the conversation. Many respected thinkers argued that life expectancy had a hard limit, so that humanity would cease to see gains going forward. One of the first to make this assertion was Louis Dublin, who in 1928 estimated that U.S. life expectancy, which was around 57 years, would never be any greater than 64.75 years.[5] He was not the first to be wrong.

According to historian Jim Oeppen and demographer James Vaupel, at least thirteen other estimates by organizations such as the United Nations and the World Bank have been made and subsequently proved inaccurate.[6] To the surprise of many, world life expectancy has more than doubled over the past two centuries, and the gains have not just been at younger ages. Oeppen and Vaupel point out that "in the second half of the 20th century, improvements in survival after age 65 propelled the rise in length of people's lives."[7] This data shouldn't be a surprise anymore. Most of us know many older people who don't actually seem old at all.

Most sixty-five-year-olds today are in much better shape than a typical sixty-five-year-old would have been in 1900. Indeed, it is not unheard of for ninety-one-year-olds like Canadian Olga Kotelko, who was profiled in the *New York Times*, to compete in athletic circuits. The *Times* reported that of the thousands who competed in a master's track championship in 2010, "hundreds were older than 75."[8] It is possible to stay healthier longer not only because of better nutrition and living conditions, but also because medical technology has advanced beyond simply fighting infectious diseases. The old are no longer quite as old as they used to be—a fact that shows up in both statistics and polls.

According to the U.S. National Long-Term Care Survey published in 2006, "Chronic disability among older Americans has dropped dramatically, and the rate of decline has accelerated during the past two decades."[9] Chronic diseases are also striking people at later ages than they used to, but perhaps most telling is how individuals respond to poll questions on the subject. According to a Pew Research Center Social and Demographic Trends survey on aging, most adults over age fifty feel at least ten years younger than their actual age, one-third of those between sixty-five and seventy-four feel ten to nineteen years younger, and one-sixth of people seventy-five and older said they felt twenty years younger. Even among those seventy-five and older, just a little more than one-third said they felt old.[10] It seems then, for many people, that "old" won't describe them until they get much older. As we shall see, this attitude is set to expand.

SCIENCE FICTION BECOMING REALITY

At thirty years old, Claudia Castillo had such a bad case of tuberculosis that the single mother had difficulty taking care of her two children. "I was coughing all the time," she said. "I couldn't walk very far and I couldn't say more than a few words at a time before becoming breathless."[11] The part of her windpipe (trachea) that attaches to her lung so was badly damaged by the disease that the only conventional option was to have her left lung removed, which carries significant risks and a high mortality rate. Fortunately for her, she was offered a new and experimental procedure, which she accepted. The plan was to grow a new windpipe in the lab with her own stem cells and then transplant it back into her body (see Figure 2.2). She agreed, and doctors proceeded to take stem cells from her bone marrow as well as cells from her lungs. They then "seeded" those cells into a donated windpipe that had previously been stripped of all of the donor's cells so that all that was left was the scaffolding, which scientists call "extracellular matrix" (ECM). Finally, the organ was incubated in the lab for three days, after which the team of doctors transplanted the new windpipe with Claudia's own cells into her body.[12] "The moment I woke after the procedure, I looked up at the doctor and he smiled and told me it had been successful," she told a reporter for the *Telegraph*. "I knew then that I had a life and a future."[13]

Ten days after the procedure, Claudia was released from the hospital. Two months later, her lung function tests were at the better end of the normal range for a young woman and she reported that she had gone dancing and swimming in the Spanish resort destination of Ibiza.[14] Months later she was still doing fine and doctors confirmed

FIGURE 2.2

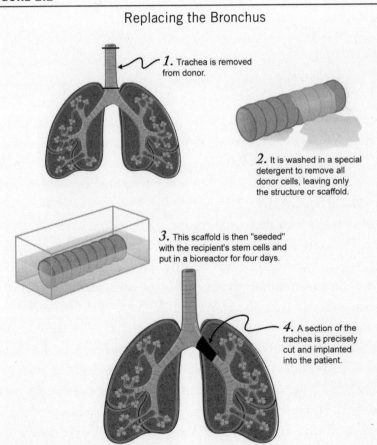

Replacing the Bronchus

1. Trachea is removed from donor.

2. It is washed in a special detergent to remove all donor cells, leaving only the structure or scaffold.

3. This scaffold is then "seeded" with the recipient's stem cells and put in a bioreactor for four days.

4. A section of the trachea is precisely cut and implanted into the patient.

SOURCE: Illustration by Paula Cruz.

that, because her own cells were used, there was no danger of her body rejecting the transplant. Clearly, Claudia's operation was a huge success. Her disease, which would have been fatal or severely disabling just years ago, has now been completely cured owing to advances in an exciting field called "tissue engineering." And growing part of a windpipe is only the beginning.

The website of the Wake Forest Institute for Regenerative Medicine introduces the world to this fascinating new technology. "Our scientists were the first in the world to successfully implant a laboratory-grown organ into humans," readers are informed, and today they "are working to grow more than 22 different organs and tissues in the laboratory."[15] Growing new hearts, livers, breast tissue, bone, and bladders are some of the many projects being spearheaded by the institute, led by the innovative Dr. Anthony Atala. Indeed, years before Claudia Castillo had ever heard of tissue engineering, Dr. Atala had already grown and implanted bladders in multiple children and teenagers suffering from a congenital birth defect that causes incomplete closure of the spine and subsequent bladder problems. Even though he pioneered the procedure in 1999, he didn't announce his results until 2006 because he wanted to make sure it worked long term. It did.

"We have shown that regenerative medicine techniques can be used to generate functional bladders that are durable," said Atala. "This suggests that regenerative medicine may one day be a solution to the shortage of donor organs in this country for those needing transplants."[16] He grew the bladders using a method similar to how Claudia's windpipe was built, but he didn't rely on a donor organ. Instead, he built a scaffold out of biodegradable materials in the shape of a bladder. He then took muscle and bladder stem cells from the patients and grew them in the lab until there were enough to place on the scaffold. He let the cells grow until the organs were ready for transplantation. Over time the scaffold degraded as the bladder tissue integrated with the body and all that was left was the new organ. As *Newsweek* reported in late 2010, Luke Masella, who was age ten when

Dr. Atala performed his procedure, is now a twenty-year-old sopho-more at the University of Connecticut and has a bladder that func-tions normally.[17] Such success stories would have sounded like science fiction twenty years ago, but they are real and augur well for the future. This is the beginning of a revolution in which we will eventually be able to replace much of our body's "hardware," including our hearts, which is encouraging because heart disease is the number one killer in the United States. No human hearts have been built yet because they are more complicated than bladders or windpipes, but that hasn't stopped innovative researchers from making great progress so far.

Dr. Doris Taylor's cardiovascular lab at the University of Min-nesota has been working on the problem and announced in 2008 that her team had managed to grow a rat heart in the lab. "When we saw the first heartbeats, we were speechless," said a member of her team.[18] As in the procedures already discussed, Taylor's lab stripped a rat heart of its cells so that all that was left was the scaffold, or the structure of the original organ. Researchers then repopulated the scaffold with cells from newborn rat hearts and coaxed the organ to beat on its own. It doesn't take a lot of imagination to predict where this research will go next. Dr. Taylor is currently repeating the ex-periment on pigs, not only because their hearts are closer in size to human hearts, but also because pig hearts are already used for re-placement parts for some human heart patients.[19]

Lungs are another incredibly complex organ, and Dr. Laura Niklason's lab at Yale University has had some success at growing and transplanting them into rats.[20] For two hours, her team's engi-neered lungs were 95 percent as efficient as natural ones. But, as in much experimental research, the process wasn't perfect. Tiny blood clots began to form, possibly because the cells weren't thick enough on the scaffold. "It's pointed out to us what worked, but it's also pointed out to us what needs to be made better," Dr. Niklason said.[21] It is not surprising that there are still issues that need to be solved before the creation of such a complex organ, but the proof of con-cept has been demonstrated—the lungs did actually work.

This chapter could be taken up just with stories of researchers all around the globe who are working on similar techniques with a variety of organs, but before we move on to look at other exciting technologies for improving human health, we should examine an alternate organ-making method that impressed editors at *Time* magazine so much that they included it in their top inventions of 2010.[22] Called "organ printing," this method is exactly what it sounds like, but instead of ink, cells are put into a printer. Likewise, instead of printing on paper, the cells are printed on a biodegradable material that operates like a scaffold. The printer then prints "pages" on top of each other in order to make a three-dimensional shape. In December 2010, a company called Organovo announced that it had successfully printed human blood vessels with its proprietary 3D printer, the NovoGen MMX Bioprinter. "These vessels are the world's first arteries made solely from cells of an individual person," said Keith Murphy, chief executive officer of Organovo.[23] Dr. Craig Kent, chief of surgery at the University of Wisconsin, added that "this is exciting progress towards functional human arterial grafts. Success in an effort like this could eventually help tens of thousands of patients."[24] Given that blood vessels are an important feature of all organs, this is the first step toward other, larger organs created in this fashion.

LEARNING FROM SALAMANDERS

The ability to rebuild body parts when people get injured or sick is something that humans have desired for millennia. Fortunately, we are finally at the point in history when this dream is starting to become reality. Aside from engineering organs, there are other methods in development to repair our bodies.

"A salamander can grow back its leg," said Dr. Atala. "Why can't a human do the same?"[25] This is a good question, and it's one that is being pursued by researchers at the McGowan Institute for Regenerative Medicine. Dr. Stephen Badylak, deputy director of the institute, has received a lot of media attention because of a material he is working with: a ground-up version of the extracellular matrix mentioned earlier, which is currently derived from pig bladders.[26] Dr. Badylak has used the ECM to grow back the tips of patients' fingers that have been accidentally snipped off, and his colleagues have used it to cure early-stage esophageal cancer by removing the cancerous cells and replacing them with the ECM.[27] Normally, after the body is injured, scarring takes place over the wound, but putting the ECM on the wound seems to prevent that from happening and also promotes new tissue growth. Scientists don't exactly understand why it works, and the ECM can't yet grow back entire limbs, but the results so far are impressive.

In one of the most recent cases, a woman named Deepa Kulkarni accidentally chopped off the tip of her pinky just above the base of her fingernail by slamming the finger in a door. When her husband took her to an emergency room, the doctors told her that there was no way to reattach the pinky and that it would be necessary to amputate even more of the finger so that it would heal properly. Deepa didn't like that prognosis and went home to scour the Internet for alternatives. That's when she found Dr. Badylak's work featured on 60 Minutes and The Oprah Winfrey Show. She emailed him out of desperation, and one of his colleagues responded the next day to say that, even though there was an alternative to amputation, they didn't know anyone in her area (Davis, California) who worked on regenerative medicine. Eventually, through emailing friends and reaching out to connections at UCLA and Berkeley, she found a local doctor who agreed to try working with the ECM, even though he hadn't done so before. Orthopedic surgeon Dr. Michael Peterson cleaned out Deepa's finger and removed the scar tissue, after which he dipped her finger into the ECM. Following seven weeks of treatment, her finger grew back, fingernail and all, and she is happy that she pushed hard to get the latest medical treatment. "Even now it's not perfect," she told CNN. "It's shorter than the other pinky, but just by looking at it you can't tell it was an amputated finger. I'm able to do everything I could do before. I wash dishes. I cook."[28]

That's a happy ending to what could have left her missing a big chunk of her finger.

Growing back parts of limbs is a step toward regrowing larger pieces, a goal of great interest to the U.S. military. Both Dr. Badylak's and Dr. Atala's organizations are supported through grants from an organization called the Armed Forces Institute of Regenerative Medicine (AFIRM). With a budget of over $250 million, AFIRM is an extremely important player pushing the field of regenerative medicine ahead.[29] Created by the U.S. Department of Defense in 2008, it was hailed as a game-changer. Dr. S. Ward Casscells, then the assistant secretary of defense for health affairs, said that "following in the great military medical tradition of innovation, collaboration and progressive research, AFIRM will unify and apply all the recent breakthroughs in regenerative medicine while leading the charge to new ones."[30] In addition to funding groups that are growing organs and salvaging limbs and digits, AFIRM is sponsoring work on burn repair, trauma repair, facial reconstruction, and scarless wound healing. ECM similar to that which helped Deepa regrow her finger also helped at least one serviceman reclaim muscle blown off in the line of duty.

Corporal Isaias Hernandez was part of a convoy in Iraq when artillery hit. Most of his colleagues died, but he escaped with wounds that included the loss of a large portion of his right thigh, which might have made amputation likely. Dr. Steven Wolf, chief of clinical trials at the U.S. Army's Institute for Surgical Research, operated on Hernandez and inserted layers of the ECM into his thigh, which spurred the growth of new muscle in a wound that had initially exposed the bone. Before the operation, Hernandez could hardly use his leg, but now he says, "I'm able to get out on my mountain bike and I can walk as far as I want."[31] His leg is not in perfect condition, but this modestly successful test case has led to clinical trials that will further explore how much muscle can be regrown.[32] "These guys, they were protecting us," Dr. Wolf said of his work on military personnel. "And from my perspective, they deserve our very best effort to do the best we know how to do, and then further, to do the best that we don't even know yet how to do."[33] The goal is clearly to grow new arms and legs when military men and women suffer trauma in battle. But will it ever really be possible? Dr. Robert Vandre, chairman of the Armed Services Biomedical Research Evaluation and Management Committee, thinks so. "Ultimately, we will be able to grow limbs," he told the American Forces Press Service.[34] That would certainly give new meaning to the slogan "Be all that you can be."

Another part of the Department of Defense working on these issues is the Defense Advanced Research Projects Agency (DARPA). The organization, which was responsible for the creation of the Internet, has its sights set on innovative technologies that could save soldiers' lives in combat. One of DARPA's projects is called "blood pharming," an attempt to secure a large supply of blood that is untainted, readily available, universal, and has a long shelf life.[35] One of the problems with treating battle wounds is that large amounts of blood can be required, but blood can stay fresh for only a limited period of time and getting fresh supplies on remote battlefields is difficult. With a $1.95 million grant from DARPA, a company called Arteriocyte created a process whereby it could generate significant amounts of blood using hematopoietic stem cells, which are derived from umbilical cord–blood units. Arteriocyte has already applied for approval from the Food and Drug Administration (FDA).[36] Although the military is a significant driver of progress in rebuilding humans, important work is also being funded through more traditional means, and one of the big breakthroughs has come from academics at a Canadian university.

MANIPULATING CELLS

On November 7, 2010, a team at McMaster University in Ontario, Canada, published work in the journal *Nature* outlining how they had turned human skin cells into blood cells in the lab.[37] Team members did it by taking samples of skin, extracting cells called fibroblasts, virally inserting a new gene (OCT4) into the cells' DNA, and then growing the cells in a mix of immune-stimulating proteins called cy-tokines. The technique was hailed as a great achievement because, unlike prior work demonstrating that skin cells could be turned into other cells, this technique did not require a middle step of returning the cells to an embryonic-like state, thereby bypassing many safety issues. Researchers made sure to replicate the process several times over two years using human skin from both young and old people in order to prove it works for a person of any age. This discovery is huge news for two reasons. First, it could mean that in the foreseeable future people needing blood for surgery, cancer treatment, or treatment of other blood conditions like anemia will be able to have blood created from a patch of their own skin to provide transfusions. McMaster University estimates that clinical trials could begin as soon as 2012.[38] And second, the technique could extend well beyond blood. It may be possible to make many types of cells out of a skin cell. "We'll now go on to work on developing other types of human cell types from skin, as we already have encouraging evidence," said Dr. Mick Bhatia, scientific director of McMaster's Stem Cell and Cancer Research Institute.[39] Being able to quickly create a specific type of cell for a patient would boost the efforts of regenerative medicine and move humanity closer to the day when replacing almost any body part when necessary will be possible.

Dr. Bhatia was working with adult cells, which clearly show great promise for therapeutic purposes. More controversial, but very powerful types of cells, are those in the embryonic stem cell category. These cells naturally have the ability to turn into any type of adult cell, and one of their success stories to date is the ability to cure spinal injuries in rats. "I have never seen in my career a biological tool as powerful as the stem cells," Dr. Hans Keirstead of UC Irvine told reporters at CBS.[40] His work, which was published in the peer-reviewed *Journal of Neuroscience* in 2005, detailed how he enabled rats with crushed spinal cords to walk again.[41] In addition to his paper, he released amazing videos of the rats before and after. First, they are crawling and unable to move their hind legs, and then after the therapy, they move around normally.[42] Dr. Keirstead explains that he was able to repair the rats by taking human embryonic cells, coaxing them into becoming cells that form myelin to protect neurons of the spinal cord, and then injecting them into the rats. This major milestone led to clinical trials in humans, with the first patient receiving treatment in October 2010 at the Shepherd Center, a spinal cord and brain injury hospital in Atlanta.[43] The human trials are being conducted by the Silicon Valley–based company Geron, and the Shepherd Center patient is the first of ten whom the company intends to enroll.

But just because the therapy worked in the animal model does not guarantee that it will work in humans, and as with any new therapy, there is always the risk that unforeseen and damaging results could occur. Also, the phase I trials will be focused only on patients who had an injury within fourteen days prior to treatment, and safety of the treatment will be Geron's first priority. That said, if ten people who were paralyzed are walking normally in a few years' time, this will prove to be yet another tool in the kit for repairing humans. And this is not the only embryonic cell trial under way. Another FDA-approved trial is being conducted by Santa Monica–based Advanced Cell Technology (ACT) and is focused on treating patients with an eye disease called Stargardt's macular dystrophy, which causes blindness, usually among youths.[44]

As we know, not all stem cell applications require embryonic cells. Dr. Bhatia's cells were created from adult skin cells but have yet to reach the trial phase. Other researchers, however, are already testing adult stem cells to treat a number of diseases. In Italy, for example, researchers were able to cure blindness in humans resulting from burns. They took stem cells from the limbus in the patient's own eye, cultured the cells, and then grafted them onto the eye. Seventy-seven percent of their patients were either cured or experienced partially restored sight. This work, which was conducted over ten years, was published in the *New England Journal of Medicine* in July 2010.[45] Other trials that have been FDA approved in the United States include using adult stem cells to treat heart disease, Lou Gehrig's disease, and limb ischemia.[46]

For those with little patience, it is frustrating to see all of this great work being conducted but not yet being made widely available to the general public. FDA trials typically take years, and as of this writing, the FDA has not approved any stem cell treatments in the United States. That, however, hasn't stopped some doctors from forging ahead in some areas. At the Centeno-Schultz Clinic in Broomfield, Colorado, doctors are using stem cell therapy to treat knee and hip pain as well as for other types of joint repair.[47] The therapy involves taking bone marrow stem cells from the patient's hip with a needle, as well as some blood. The samples are then sent to the lab for processing and then are reinjected into the area in need of repair using imaging guidance. Doctors at the clinic have published studies showing that the therapy works in terms of both boosting cartilage and reducing pain.[48] They note that they were able to help professional football player Jarvis Green, whose failed knee surgery contributed to his missing games and being let go by the Denver Broncos. Following the procedure, called Regenexx, Green was picked up by the Houston Texans, passed a team physician physical, and "states that he was able to try out in full form without limitations."[49] "If I didn't do the stem cell treatments, I wouldn't have a job," Green said. "Before the therapy I had trouble even getting in and out of the car, and now I have no worries. You can see that my knees have improved by looking at the MRI. My quality of life is much better and I have the chance to keep playing football. We all have guardian angels."[50] The doctors claim that they are able to offer the treatments without FDA approval because a patient's own stem cells are not a drug and therefore fall outside of FDA jurisdiction.[51] The FDA has taken the opposite position, and the issue will be settled by the courts.[52]

MANIPULATING GENES

Gene therapy, the process of modifying genes by adding new DNA or turning off parts of existing DNA, has been hailed by some as the "holy grail" of bioengineering. Although this field stalled about a decade ago after children who were part of early trials died, procedures have become better over time as researchers learn more about how to safely introduce new DNA into the body.[53] One of the problems with gene therapy is that it can be difficult to insert a new gene exactly where scientists want it to go because altered viruses are often used as the carriers for new genetic information and they will attach themselves to whatever spot in the host's genome that they can find. A second problem is that some viruses, such as the adenovirus, create an inflammatory response. One method to counter this problem is to use a different virus, such as the stealthy adeno-associated virus, which does not normally stimulate an immune response. That was the technique used to cure nine-year-old Corey Haas, who suffered from a hereditary blindness called leber congenital amaurosis (LCA).

When he was a baby, Corey's parents noticed that he would often drop items right in front of himself but not be able to see them to pick them up. Worried, they took him to a doctor and learned that he was legally blind because of a genetic mutation that had left his body unable to make certain proteins needed for proper sight. Then, they did what most loving parents would do: they searched for a solution. What they found was a gene therapy trial at the Children's Hospital of Philadelphia. Led by Dr. Katherine A. High, the research team injected into Corey's eye a "transgene"—a genetically engineered virus that carried a normal version of the gene that is mutated in people with LCA (see Figure 2.3).[54] The treatment was a stunning success. Corey's body started producing the proteins that he had previously lacked, and his world changed for the better. "His independence has increased, and he's able to play like a normal child now," his father told the press.[55] It's truly a wonderful outcome for a young boy with the rest of his life ahead of him.

Even though gene therapy for LCA appears to be a huge success, there is still a long way to go before gene therapy can live up to early expectations. For instance, although Italian and Israeli researchers reported in January 2009 that gene therapy cured eight of ten children who were suffering from "bubble boy" disease, otherwise known as

FIGURE 2.3

How It Works

Using DNA, scientists create a functioning gene to replace the faulty one in the retina. Then they place the new gene inside a little "coat" made up of viral proteins (known as a vector). The type of virus researchers use does not have the ability to reproduce or cause disease.

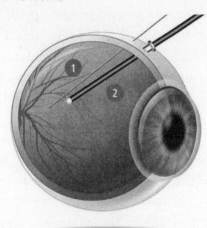

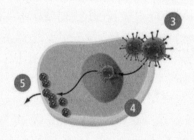

Scientists add in the new gene by injecting it directly into the eye (above) through a thin needle (1) connected to a syringe, with the help of a light probe (2). The new gene (3) enters the cell nucleus (4), where it makes the healthy enzymes (5) required to see.

SOURCE: "One Shot of Gene Therapy and Children with Congenital Blindness Can Now See," Children's Hospital of Philadelphia, October 24, 2009, http://multivu.prnewswire .com/mnr/chop/40752/. Illustration courtesy of the Children's Hospital of Philadelphia.

severe combined immunodeficiency, the treatment was not problem-free. The inherited disease causes nonfunctional immune systems, which means that without advanced treatment, these children die in their first year of life. That eight patients were able to develop functional immune systems through the therapy is impressive, but the serious side effects included hypertension and autoimmune hepatitis, among others.[56] Likewise, gene therapy for late-stage skin cancer was able to wipe out the disease, but only in two of seventeen patients treated by Dr. Steven Rosenberg at the U.S. National Cancer Institute.[57] When asked about the difficulties in this type of work, Dr. Rosenberg replied, "We've used viruses to introduce new genes into cells to make them into cancer-fighting cells, and we can do it much better two years later. So, my hope is, as we continue to improve this technology, the response rates are going to go up."[58]

One new technique that promises to make gene therapy more precise goes by the name "zinc finger nucleases."[59] Used by the body to turn genes on and off, zinc fingers are proteins attached with an ion of zinc that holds them together in a "finger"-like manner. When fused with a nuclease (an enzyme that cuts DNA), they have the ability to precisely edit DNA by binding to a set of three letters of DNA code, and with just six fingers scientists can attach to any particular gene. Much of the intellectual property surrounding zinc fingers, discovered by British crystallographer Aaron Klug, is owned by California biotech company Sangamo BioSciences.[60] At the time of this writing, a human clinical trial using zinc finger nucleases was being conducted by Dr. Carl June at the University of Pennsylvania to fight AIDS. In phase 1 of the safety trial, Dr. June removed some of the patient's T cells (those normally attacked by HIV), used a zinc finger nuclease to disable the CCR5 gene that HIV attaches to, and then cultured the cells and injected them back into the patient's body. The results showed that the new T cells were tolerated by the body and multiplied.[61] This is exciting because there is only one case of someone ever being cured of HIV (Timothy Brown has been HIV free since 2008), which was the result of a bone marrow treatment from a person resistant to AIDS owing to a natural mutation in the CCR5 gene (the percentage of people with this resistance is very small).[62] And while the race continues to make gene therapy safer and more effective, researchers using animal models show that great possibilities await.

THE PLASTICITY OF AGING

Gene therapy has been shown to reverse type 1 diabetes in mice, speed muscle healing, and achieve other results. But perhaps the most interesting animal studies involve those that extend healthy life span. Dr. Cynthia Kenyon of the University of California, San Francisco, has become well known for her discovery that partially disabling a single gene, called daf-2, doubled the life of tiny worms called *Caenorhabditis elegans*.[63] Her lab later noted that altering the daf-16 gene and other cells added to the impact, allowing the worms to survive in a healthy state six times longer than their normal life span. In human terms, they would be the equivalent of healthy, active five-hundred-year-olds.[64]

Experiments in animal models are not always applicable to humans, but humans do have the same sort of pathways that Dr. Kenyon manipulated, so similar genetic techniques may one day allow us to live longer in a healthier state as well. As Dr. Kenyon explained, "Our discoveries have led to the realization that the aging process, like everything else in biology, is under exquisite regulation, in this case, by a complex, multifaceted hormonal and transcriptional system that affects aging in many species, including mammals."[65] This regulation can clearly be altered, making aging, once thought to be a process set in stone, malleable. Indeed, Dr. Kenyon acknowledged this fact, noting, "People have always thought that, like a car, our body parts eventually wear out. But we found that over time, when one gene was manipulated, the worm actually remained youthful—in all ways—so that age-related diseases were also postponed."[66]

This reality has been confirmed by the work of many other researchers. For instance, Dr. Robert J. Shmookler Reis's laboratory at the University of Arkansas managed to genetically alter worms to live ten times longer than normal.[67] Likewise, Dr. Maria Blasco of Spain's National Cancer Research Center found an altogether different way to extend the lives of mice by 45 percent. Dr. Blasco's team turned up the gene that affects production of an enzyme called telomerase, which helps to keep the ends of chromosomes from shortening, thereby allowing cells to keep replicating. But because cells that keep replicating often cause cancer, her team also engineered the mice to be cancer resistant by adding the genes p53, p16, and p19ARF.[68] The result, published in the peer-reviewed journal *Cell*, was radically extended healthy life spans for some lucky mice. If humans were to increase their life expectancy by 45 percent, they could live to around 116 years old.

THE SEARCH FOR AN ANTIAGING PILL

Aside from gene therapy, other ideas for increasing healthy life span include various pharmaceuticals or compounds. Perhaps the one that has made the biggest splash from a public awareness point of view is resveratrol, a type of polyphenol found in the skins of red grapes and red wine. In 2006 Harvard professor David Sinclair's lab discovered that at high doses resveratrol protected mice from the ill health effects of a high-fat diet, such as diabetes and heart disease.[69] This work was encouraging because scientists already knew that resveratrol could extend the life spans of yeast, flies, worms, and fish. It appeared that the same effects were likely for larger animals. Science writer David Stipp recounts how he was surprised at how effective the compound seemed to be. "After watching elderly mice on resveratrol perform like rodent Olympians in an endurance test, I came away convinced that the long, weird quest to extend life span . . . was finally getting somewhere."[70]

Resveratrol affects a set of enzymes called sirtuins, which are known to be involved in the proven life-span-extension method called caloric restriction (CR). CR is exactly what it sounds like: eating about 30 percent fewer calories than normal but without malnutrition. It is well documented that CR causes an extension in both health and life span in rodents, delaying the onset of age-related diseases such as cancer, heart disease, and Alzheimer's. The evidence shows that even in monkeys CR is powerful. In 2009 results from a twenty-year-long study on caloric restriction in rhesus monkeys demonstrated the health effects.[71] The monkeys on the low-calorie diet not only were in better health and suffered fewer deaths than the control group but also looked a lot better. The passage of time was tougher on the regular monkeys than on the calorie-restricted ones (see Figure 2.4).

Of course, few people are willing to restrict their calories by 30 percent, so there was much excitement when news reports suggested that Dr. Sinclair had found a compound that could mimic the effects of CR. Dr. Sinclair's company, Sirtris Pharmaceuticals, was sold to GlaxoSmithKline in 2008 for $720 million, and clinical trials began on "small molecule drugs" that, like resveratrol, affect sirtuins. As of

FIGURE 2.4

Animal Appearance in Old Age
(A–B) Photographs of a typical control animal at
27.6 years of age (~age of average life span).
(C–D) Photographs of an age-matched animal on CR.

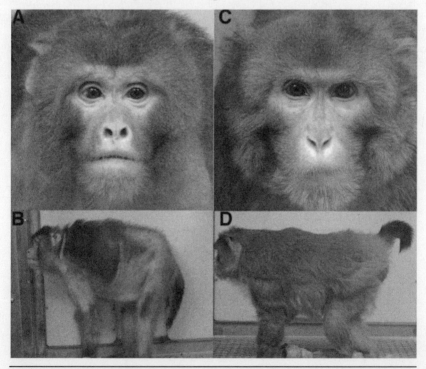

Source: National Institutes of Health, www.ncbi.nlm.nih.gov/pmc/articles/PMC2812 811/figure/F1/. R. J. Colman, R. M. Anderson et al., "Caloric Restriction Delays Disease Onset and Mortality in Rhesus Monkeys," *Science,* July 10, 2009. Reprinted with permission from the American Association for the Advancement of Science (AAAS).

this writing, phase 1 trials for one of Sirtris's drugs showed that it was safe, but there is no word yet on how well it might work in humans.[72] Additional studies done by the National Institute on Aging indicate that resveratrol alone did not extend life in healthy mice, although it did protect the obese ones, so for now resveratrol itself does not seem to be the panacea everyone had hoped. It is possible that Dr. Sinclair's team will fare better with proprietary compounds, particularly if they target them to treat diseases like diabetes.[73] As Dr. Sinclair told the *New York Times* in 2006, "The goal is not just to make people live longer. It's to see eventually that an 80-year-old feels like a 50-year-old does today."[74]

Another pharmaceutical-based story to make big news was that of rapamycin, a drug that has traditionally been used to keep the body from rejecting organ and bone marrow transplants. It has fared slightly better than resveratrol in mouse studies, and perhaps the most promising finding involving this drug was the discovery that aging can be regulated even when the therapy is initiated at older ages. In a study published in *Nature*, researchers demonstrated that they were able to extend the lives and health of mice by 14 percent for females and 9 percent for males even when the drug was administered when they were six hundred days old, the equivalent of a sixty-year-old human.[75] Most scientists agree that there is no clear way to translate these results into a therapy for humans, but it is proof of concept for at least two important notions: that one molecule can have a huge impact on aging and that interventions late in life can slow aging.

One last compound that we will consider in this chapter is TA-65, a telomerase activator discovered by Geron and licensed to a company called T.A. Sciences. Telomeres are the protective caps at the ends of chromosomes in cells. Chromosomes contain our genetic information. Every time a healthy cell divides, the telomeres get a little shorter. Dr. Elizabeth Blackburn, who won the Nobel Prize in 2009 for her co-discovery of how chromosomes are protected by telomeres, says that we can think of telomeres "like the tips of shoelaces. If you lose the tips, the ends start fraying."[76] Telomerase is an enzyme that restores the length of the telomeres as they wear down. TA-65 is thought to stimulate more of this enzyme, with the hope that if telomeres stay longer, the aging process won't move ahead quite so fast. So far there is no solid proof that this idea is correct, but there are a number of people who have been willing to pay the $1,200 to $4,000 price for a six-month supply of the supplement, and T.A. Sciences published a study in the peer-reviewed journal *Rejuvenation Research* showing that TA-65 did activate the enzyme telomerase in one hundred volunteer subjects over one year (although there was no control group).[77] Whether this supplement will actually help those who take it live longer and healthier lives is still up for vigorous debate. Some scientists even warn that taking the compound could lead to serious problems over the long run because stimulating telomerase in mice has been shown to raise the risk of cancer.[78] To counter these types of worries, the company notes, "TA-65 has been in use since 2005 with not one reported adverse event."[79] Given that T.A. Sciences has a fairly large group of volunteers taking this product, it will be interesting to see if that claim holds up over the long run.

GREATEST ENGINEERING PROJECT OF ALL TIME

It should be clear by now that the aging process can be manipulated and humans can be repaired in multiple ways. These facts lead to one logical conclusion: that engineering the human body is one of the greatest projects of all time. Aside from the important work that has resulted in creating replacement body parts, altering genes, and better understanding aging, there is another huge reason to be optimistic about the prospects of rebuilding humans when they get sick: the ability to sequence the human genome, or the complete set of human DNA.

The Human Genome Project (HGP), which was coordinated by the U.S. Department of Energy and the National Institutes of Health (NIH), kick-started this field. Francis Collins, now the director of the NIH, was the leader of the HGP, which set as its goal to sequence all the DNA in the human body. On June 26, 2000, the first draft of the human blueprint was announced at the White House. "Humankind is on the verge of gaining immense new power to heal. Genome science . . . will revolutionize the diagnosis, prevention and treatment of most, if not all, human diseases," President Bill Clinton announced.[80] Understanding the building blocks of an organism increases the possibility of reverse-engineering and rebuilding that organism, so President Clinton's enthusiasm was well placed even if such understanding is taking longer than most hoped. And once it became clear that the human body has a "source code" that can be altered, it didn't take long for engineers to become much more interested in biology. There exists a software program for the body; the key now is to figure out how to rewrite or hack it.

Of course, even though the HGP was officially completed in 2003, our understanding of how the human genome works is still in its infancy, and we continue to learn about new aspects of the system.[81] One of the things that will speed up this understanding is faster and cheaper sequencing capabilities. Because advances in computing continue to expand exponentially, it won't be long before affordable and fast sequencing will be widespread. Consider that whereas the Human Genome Project cost roughly $2.7 billion, in 2007 it cost about $2 million to sequence James Watson's genome, and by 2009 Complete Genomics said it would be able to sequence an entire human genome for around $5,000, assuming a bulk order of forty or more genomes.[82] That's quite a reduction in costs in only a few years' time. Some scientists in London have even predicted that they will eventually be able to do it "for a few dollars."[83] Whatever the final price, eventually genome sequencing will be so fast and cheap that everyone will be able to do it, a boon to researchers trying to understand how the body works and, ultimately, how to fight disease. Even with today's high prices, sequencing has led to some useful information.

One of the first successes came in 2005 when researchers discovered that age-related macular degeneration, which causes blindness in older people, was associated with a gene that was seemingly unrelated to vision. "No one had previously suspected that particular gene, which plays a role in inflammation," wrote Dr. Collins. "This underscores the power of researchers being able to scan the whole genome, and not just limit their searches to their own best hunches."[84] This power also translates into discovering weaknesses in cancer cells, thereby making possible personalized treatment, as well as looking at the genomes of people who live a very long time to see if they possess certain protector genes that regular people do not.

There are at least two well-known groups studying centenarians (people who are older than one hundred). One is the Boston University New England Centenarian Study, run by Dr. Thomas Perls, and the other is the Longevity Genes Project at the Albert Einstein College of Medicine, run by Dr. Nir Barzilai. According to Dr. Perls's research, even though lifestyle and habits are important for health, it is clear that "exceptional longevity runs very strongly in families."[85] Dr. Nir Barzilai agrees. The "super agers," as he calls them, appear to have a heritable genetic makeup that allows them to better avoid cardiovascular disease, insulin resistance, and high blood pressure.[86] The key, of course, is to find out exactly what parts of their genetic code keep them so healthy. Once more genomes are sequenced and our understanding advances, it may be possible to design genetic therapies to fight aging. And if the human source code can be altered, then so can the code of any living organism.

Dr. Craig Venter, whose company Celera Genomics competed with the government-funded HGP, was also given credit for being first to sequence the human genome. He has since moved on to other projects and in May 2010 announced that his group was the first to create a synthetic cell. We will learn more about this milestone in Chapter 8, but the important point is that biology has been turned into an information technology. "In essence, scientists are digitizing biology by converting the A, C, T, and G's of the chemical makeup of DNA into 1's and 0's in a computer," Dr. Venter's institute explains on its website.[87] And Dr. Venter is not the only one to look at things this way. DARPA has disclosed that it is backing the biology-as-engineering outlook with $6 million on a project called "bio-design" and $20 million for synthetic biology. As a *Wired News* article puts it, "DARPA is looking to re-write the laws of evolution to the military's advantage, creating 'synthetic organisms' that can live forever—or can be killed with the flick of a molecular switch."[88]

Synthetic biology has many implications, but for those concerned with extending human health span, Dr. Aubrey de Grey offers what he believes is a comprehensive road map to fighting aging. A computer scientist turned gerontologist, de Grey believes that there are seven different ways to engineer around the damage that aging inflicts on our bodies, which collectively may deliver comprehensive regenerative medicine against aging. He calls his plan Strategies for Engineered Negligible Senescence (SENS), and his outline of how each strategy could be implemented is detailed in his book *Ending Aging: The Rejuvenation Breakthroughs That Could Reverse Human Aging in Our Lifetime*.[89] An example of one of his engineering suggestions is to insert enzymes into the body's lysosomes (little cellular recycling centers) in order to make them better at eliminating the "junk" that builds up in cells over time. This would help fight aging because when too much junk builds up, the cells die. Table 2.1 contains a short summary of his very complex plan.

Most nonscientist eyes will glaze over when looking at this chart, but it is based on a detailed review of an enormous body of scientific literature. And so far no one has been able to show that de Grey is off base in his proposal, even though in July 2005 the MIT Technology Review challenged scientists to disprove his claims, offering a $20,000 prize to any molecular biologist who could demonstrate that "SENS is so wrong that it is unworthy of learned debate."[90] As de Grey is happy to point out, the challenge remains open. Indeed, he argues that there is much room for optimism because "for each major aging lesion, a SENS solution for its removal or repair either already exists in prototype form, or is foreseeable from existing scientific developments."[91] This optimism has led him to make the provocative claim that the

TABLE 2.1

The Seven Major Classes of Cellular and Molecular Damage
According to SENS

Aging Damage	Discovery	SENS Solution
Cell loss, tissue atrophy	1955	Stem cells and tissue engineering (RepleniSENS)
Nuclear [epi]mutations (only cancer matters)	1959, 1982	Removal of telomere-lengthening machinery (OncoSENS)
Mutant mitochondria	1972	Allotopic expression of 13 proteins (MitoSENS)
Death-resistant cells	1965	Targeted ablation (ApoptoSENS)
Tissue stiffening	1958, 1981	AGE-breaking molecules (GlycoSENS); tissue engineering
Extracellular aggregates	1907	Immunotherapeutic clearance (AmyloSENS)
Intracellular aggregates	1959	Novel lysosomal hydrolases (LysoSENS)

SOURCE: Based on data provided by SENS Foundation, "Research Themes," www.sens
.org/sens-research/research-themes.

first humans to live to 1,000 years may have already been born. Such
a statement seems far-fetched to many, but so did the idea of growing
an organ before it was actually done. Only time will tell whether humans will ever reach four-digit age brackets, but we undoubtedly have
entered a period in which our scientific capabilities will allow us to
repair ourselves and engineer longer life expectancies with better
health. It is therefore not at all radical to consider a future where humans might enjoy one-hundred-plus birthdays, more predictably and
in greater shape than ever before.

In this chapter, we have seen how life expectancy has grown dramatically over time, but that growth is only the beginning. Now that
biology has become an engineering project, we can expect many more

advances to help extend life expectancy, even at older ages. Tissue engineering, gene therapy, and stem cells, combined with a clear understanding that aging is plastic and can be altered, place us at an important turning point in history. That the human genome has been identified and sequencing techniques are getting faster and more affordable will allow for a better understanding of disease and the potential manipulation of DNA to repair problems, even before they occur. Complicated engineering proposals with the goal of avoiding aging already exist and are challenging scientists to implement them. It is unclear just how long humans will be able to extend their health spans, but few dispute it will happen. This book assumes that human life expectancy will one day reach 150 years and that health span will extend along with it. Some scientists would say that is a conservative estimate based on the possibilities, but it is radical enough to change our social, economic, and cultural worlds. The next chapter, then, will take a look at the explosive question of population growth and the environment in a longer-lived world.

CHAPTER 3

Mother Nature and the Longevity Revolution

T HE NEXT TIME you're at a cocktail party, try asking the other guests what a Stanford University aeronautics student has in common with a farmer in Illinois. If no one can guess, try making the question easier by asking what a United Airlines 737 jet and a John Deere tractor have in common. The answer is a precision global positioning system (GPS).

Tractors have come a long way since manufacturer John Deere started out in 1837 forging his first steel plow. If Deere were alive today, he would certainly be surprised to see tractors help drive themselves. Indeed, farming is not an occupation that springs to mind when one thinks about GPS. Yet in 1993 Michael O'Connor, then a PhD student at Stanford, realized that the GPS he was working with could be used to save farmers money by reducing waste.

"Back then, GPS was not a household name," O'Connor recalls. "My parents said, 'Mike, you work on the craziest things.'"[1] But his strange-sounding idea turned into a huge benefit, not only for farmers but also for the environment and consumers.

When farmers work their fields, they go back and forth over many hectares for hours at a time. If they don't drive in perfectly parallel lines, or if they drive over the same area twice, these deviations can cost thousands of dollars in wasted fuel, fertilizer, and pesticides. O'Connor led a team that invented a system called AutoFarm, sold by Novariant, that prevents these problems. With GPS precisely guiding a tractor, combine, or harvester to within three centimeters of a specified path, there is less waste and fewer pollutants from the burning of fossil fuel, overuse of fertilizer, or bulk spraying of pesticide. Not surprisingly, farmers give the system glowing reviews.

According to custom planter David Braga of Caruthers, California, AutoFarm not only helps with creating efficient rows but also makes the actual work much quicker. "I planted 200 acres in rolling hills in Yuba City this spring in 24 hours," he told *Western Farm Press*. "Before GPS that would take four or five days."[2]

Braga made this comment in 2000 when the first GPS tractors were just hitting the market. Since then the technology has gotten better and more refined as Novariant and similar competing companies have worked with farmers to improve the technology. "Every one year to 18 months we introduce something new," O'Connor reported in 2009.[3]

These efficiency gains pay off in terms of fewer pollutants, greater revenue, and higher yields. For instance, if a California tomato grower were able to add 2 percentage points to his or her yield by eliminating "guess rows," the spaces in between rows that can be too big owing to the driver guessing, an additional twenty acres would be farmable. This would result in an additional $40,000 in revenue and a whole lot more tomatoes for consumers to eat.[4]

Why does this tractor example matter for a book about longevity? Because it helps to demonstrate how human ingenuity works to solve real and potential problems, such as food shortages, that might occur if longevity leads to increased population growth. In 2008 John Deere's then-CEO Robert W. Lane discussed how he sees a bright future for similar advances.

"Every indication is that the dramatic increase in yield, which we've already experienced, will continue and maybe even accelerate," Lane told *Fortune* magazine. "We are at a huge transition to intelligent machinery, from planting and spraying to harvesting at the optimal time to fewer chemicals being applied to much smarter use of seeds."[5]

Indeed, it is the ingenuity of people like Michael O'Connor and the folks at John Deere who were motivated to improve the human condition that led to the massive increases in life expectancy in developed countries in the first place. As we learned in the previous chapter, advances in nutrition, sanitation, technologies, and medicine were responsible for the longer lives we now enjoy, particularly in the Western world. This is great news, yet one of the outcomes of this reality is population growth—an issue that worries many.

THE EARTH'S ABILITY TO
HANDLE LONGER-LIVED HUMANS

Increased health and life spans may be a dream come true, but many worry that it could turn nightmarish owing to problems like overcrowding, resource depletion, and greater pollution. Living a long time might be wonderful on an individual basis, but if many people can do it, would the world still be a place in which we would want to reside? This is a legitimate worry because both the U.S. and world populations continue to grow.

For instance, in 1800 America's population totaled just over 5 million—that's fewer people than currently live in New York City. By 2011 that number had grown to over 311 million.[6] Likewise, the world population in 1800 was estimated at around 900 million and by early 2011 the U.S. Census World POPClock estimated that number at 6.8 billion.[7] Of course, during that time the economy changed and living conditions improved significantly, driving up life expectancy by decades. Nevertheless, 6.8 billion is a big number. Can the planet and our societal structures handle any more people?

This chapter will take at close look at three core concerns with the longevity revolution: population growth, potential scarcity of resources, and pollution that larger numbers of people could cause.

MODELING POPULATIONS
WITH LONGER LIVES

This book considers a world in which humans will live to 150 years in a healthy state—almost a doubling of current life expectancy. People who would have become sick and passed away at sixty, seventy, or eighty will have their healthy lives extended. If fertility rates remain similar to what they are today, then populations around the world will expand. But by how much?

Because the legitimate possibility of significant life extension at older ages is a new development, estimates of population growth from the usual places, such as the United Nations or the World Bank, are not available. However, a team of scholars at the University of Chicago has been thinking about such ideas and has worked out a model that it has used to analyze data for Sweden, a favorite for demographers because of its long data sets. When compared to the rest of Europe, Sweden also happens to have relatively high fertility and low mortality.

After calculating various longevity scenarios using a type of model similar to that of the World Bank and other countries, Dr. Leonid Gavrilov and Dr. Natalia Gavrilova concluded that even if humans completely stopped aging and essentially became immortal, Sweden's population would increase by only 22 percent over one hundred years. "Population changes are surprisingly slow in their response to dramatic life extension," they wrote in a study published in the journal *Rejuvenation Research*.[8] Without any life extension, Sweden's population, which in 2005 was just over 9 million, is set to decline to around 6 million in one hundred years. The Gavrilovs did not calculate what the population increase would be if the Swedes merely extended their time by 70 years (to 150 years), but given that extending it indefinitely would cause only a 22 percent increase, it is safe to say that 70 years wouldn't move the dial by much. One of the reasons that cutting death rates doesn't affect population as much as we might think is that heavy population growth really comes from births, not from fewer deaths. In countries like Sweden, where the fertility rate in 2005 was 1.8, each pair of parents isn't replacing themselves. And fertility rates are expected to continue their decline as countries continue to build wealth.

Indeed, while overall population is still growing, the *rate* at which it is growing is actually slowing down (see Figure 3.1).[9] Even though the UN population projection for the year 2050 is 9.2 billion, fertility rates are expected to decline from 2.55 children per woman today to 2.02 children per woman for *all* women in the world, including those in developing countries. Of course, that projection is based on what the world looks like *today*. Once we reach the point at which people realize that they will be living significantly longer themselves, the fertility rates may change.

Historically, as people became wealthier and better educated, two aspects positively correlated with greater longevity, they tended to have fewer children. Speaking from his experience with the Gates

FIGURE 3.1

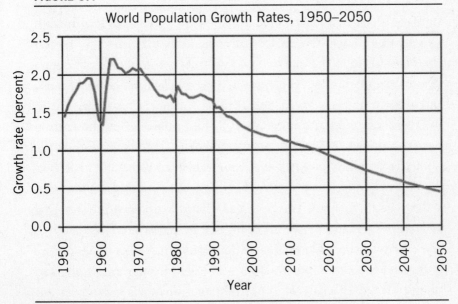

World Population Growth Rates, 1950–2050

SOURCE: U.S. Census Bureau, International Database, December 2010.

Foundation, Bill Gates notes, "In places like Thailand and Bangladesh, it has already been shown that, with proper education and adequate medical care, people choose to have a number of children that their family can support."[10] Even though this is certainly true, some research now suggests that the trend of fertility decline associated with wealth may actually be one side of a J-shaped curve, with fertility going back up as people become even wealthier.[11] If this turns out to be true, the "rule" that richer societies have fewer children may be wrong over the long run. It is difficult to predict what will happen to fertility rates in the future, and depending on which rate is factored into the assumptions, the United Nations notes that the world population could either grow or shrink.[12] If we take a middle ground and assume moderate population growth owing to decreased fertility rates and increased longevity, then we should next consider whether we would have the resources needed for these additional people.

WHY THOMAS MALTHUS WAS WRONG

In his *Essay on the Principle of Population* (1798), Thomas Malthus advanced this thesis: "The power of population is indefinitely greater than the power in the earth to produce subsistence for man. Population, when unchecked, increases in a geometrical ratio. Subsistence increases only in an arithmetical ratio. A slight acquaintance with numbers will show the immensity of the first power in comparison with the second."[13] This notion that population grows faster than the ability to provide for ourselves seems intuitive to some and was borrowed by Stanford professor Paul Ehrlich, who wrote the 1968 best-selling eco-doom book *The Population Bomb*. Ehrlich was so sure that humans were going to overpopulate that he predicted, "In the 1970s the world will undergo famines—hundreds of millions of people are going to starve to death in spite of any crash programs embarked upon now. At this late date nothing can prevent a substantial increase in the world death rate, although many lives could be saved through dramatic programs to stretch the carrying capacity of the earth by increasing food production."[14]

Instead, the opposite happened. Today, many around the world are struggling with obesity, or the consumption of too much food, all while the world's population has been growing (see Figure 3.2). Since 1800 the price of wheat has been steadily declining and the daily intake of calories per capita in *both* the developed and developing countries has been on the rise.[15]

FIGURE 3.2

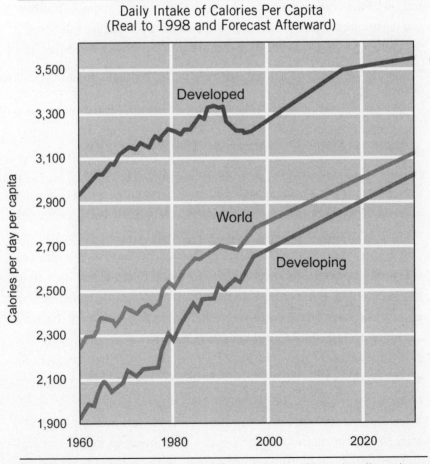

Daily Intake of Calories Per Capita
(Real to 1998 and Forecast Afterward)

SOURCE: Bjorn Lomborg, Director of Copenhagen Consensus Center, http://copenhagen.com.

The explanation for this seemingly strange outcome was nicely summed up by Julian Simon when he told *Wired* magazine, "Human beings create more than they use, on average. It had to be so, or we would be an extinct species."[16] To flesh out this statement, let's look at more of the facts and at a rather famous bet between Ehrlich and Simon on the matter.

After Paul Ehrlich made the apocalyptic claim that "if I were a gambler, I would take even money that England will not exist in the year 2000," Simon suggested a wager on a less ridiculous idea: that "the cost of non-government-controlled raw materials (including grain and oil) will not rise in the long run."[17] Simon was concerned with *long-run* prices because that is a better way to gauge real trends. For the purposes of this book, the long run is extremely important because life extension means that the long run will matter even more, not less.

Ehrlich accepted the bet and chose five metals that he thought would rise in price as they became scarce owing to human population growth.[18] During the decade from 1980 to 1990, world population grew more than 800 million—a huge increase that, according to Ehrlich, should have spelled disaster. So what happened to the price of metals during this population boom? Without fail, every single metal decreased in price, and Ehrlich was forced to admit defeat.[19]

Now, one might think that Simon just got lucky and that the decade from 1980 to 1990 happened to be one of decreases in metals prices, but that isn't the case. Research since 1990 shows that, despite ups and downs, the overall trend in these prices is downward. Indeed, according to David McClintick and Ross B. Emmett in an article for the Property and Environment Research Center, "a wager in 1900 would have been won in 1999 by the person who predicted a decrease in natural resource prices. If someone invested $200 at 1900 metals' prices in each of these five metals the inflation-adjusted value of the same bundle of metals in 1999 would have been 53 percent lower. The person who took Simon's position would have won over the entire century."[20] And this decline in prices happened while the world population grew during the course of the century by an immense 4.4 billion people.[21] What this example demonstrates is the counterintuitive reality that greater numbers of humans do not necessarily translate into fewer resources on which to live.

Simon's work prompted the National Academy of Sciences to explore the issue more carefully.[22] The resulting book, titled *Population Growth and Economic Development*, explained that "concern about the impact of rapid population growth on resource exhaustion has often been exaggerated" and that market adaptations "serve to greatly mute, and perhaps entirely counteract, any negative effect of resource depletion on the standard of living."[23] Many scholars have reached the same conclusion, and University of Pennsylvania demography professor Samuel Preston goes so far as to say that "as a simple collection of mass, the human population has no environmental implications." He notes that if a population of 5.6 billion humans stood together, they "would occupy a circle with a radius of less than 8 miles that extended an infinitesimal distance into the atmosphere."[24] That is, it is not just *numbers* of humans, but their *activity* that matters. Nevertheless, such a conclusion might seem hard to understand until we realize that more people mean *more ideas*.

In an interview with the *Wall Street Journal*'s Paul Hofheinz, Microsoft cofounder Bill Gates explained the dynamic this way: "Malthus was wrong because his math didn't adequately take into account the influence and power of the human mind."[25] That is, more ideas lead to new ways of producing the things that we need, which is why we are not facing scarcity even in the face of population growth. We can also look at the issue from the genius perspective. According to Mensa International, only 2 percent of the population are geniuses, so for every 100,000 people, there are 2,000 brilliant people.[26] Each of those people can be only so creative, so if their numbers are doubled, so, too, are the opportunities for new and innovative ideas. Of course, one doesn't need to be a Mensa-qualified genius to come up with interesting ways to make the world a better place, but the example helps to show why more people can actually lead to improved conditions.

For a more concrete example of how Simon's belief in human creativity paid off, we can think about the metal copper, which has many
uses, one of them being telephone infrastructure. Back in 1980 copper
wires were the key ingredient for America's telecommunications
network, making copper quite expensive because demand seemed
only to be growing. Such facts convinced Paul Ehrlich to select it as a
commodity that he thought would grow in both scarcity and price. Increasing numbers of people would certainly require more infrastructure, and therefore more copper would seem to be required. Indeed,
the fact that in 1979 telephone company AT&T owned the biggest
untapped copper mine in the world suggested that even private business was betting on copper continuing to grow in scarcity and hence
in material value. So what happened to make the price of copper drop
a mere ten years later?

First, the price of copper did go up in response to market scarcity,
sending a strong signal to the market that replacements for its use
were needed. Second, by 1989 a solution to this price increase was
found. That year Canada's *Globe and Mail* newspaper wrote an interesting story on a copper replacement it called "Wonder Wire." The
story explained how glass strands that transmit laser light, otherwise
known as fiber optics technology, were set to overtake copper as the
main infrastructure for communications. This was the case, the newspaper wrote, because "the cost of manufacturing and installing fibre
optics lines is now almost as low as copper and may go even lower, because the price of copper is rising while that of sand, the raw material
used to make optical fibres, is not."[27]

Fiber optics are also much faster and more versatile than copper,
so copper wires for communications technology were soon thought
of as somewhat antique. Of course, the fiber optics market hit a bit
of a bump in 1999, and there are now many competing ways to provide communications services, including wireless, voice over Internet using cable, satellite, and DSL Internet technology.

What the story of copper helps to illustrate is how rising prices
caused by high demand led humans to compensate with alternatives.

It follows, then, that if food supplies became more expensive owing to increased population growth in longer-lived societies, then this higher demand would lead to alternative ways of farming aimed at producing more food. Such a revolution has already taken place to some extent in agriculture through the use of both conventional plant-breeding techniques and newer genetically engineered crops. Norman Borlaug, plant breeder and winner of the Nobel Peace Prize in 1970, is known for having reversed food shortages in India and Pakistan in the 1960s. He did this by helping to develop high-yield dwarf wheat, which has short stalks so that plants expend less energy on growing inedible stalks and more on growing grain. The result was hundreds of thousands of lives saved, perhaps even 1 billion, according to the American Council on Science and Health.[28] Research like this continues, and now scientists are focusing on how to produce higher yields with lower inputs of critical elements such as water.

Indeed, one of the biggest environmental concerns today is the depletion of freshwater supplies. According to molecular biologist and Hoover Institute fellow Henry Miller, "Agriculture accounts for about 70% of the world's freshwater consumption—and more in areas of intensive farming and arid or semi-arid conditions, such as in California. So the introduction of plants that grow with less water would free up much of that essential resource for other uses."[29] As we might expect in a time of worry about water shortages, plant biologists are already tackling this problem. Plants that can grow in lower-quality water or salty water are one response. For instance, Dr. Eduardo Blumwald at the University of California, Davis created a tomato that is often considered the first truly salt-tolerant crop, meaning that it can be grown in saline conditions yet still tastes like a regular tomato.[30] "Since environmental stress due to salinity is one of the most serious factors limiting the productivity of crops, this innovation will have significant implications for agriculture worldwide," he said when announcing his research back in 2001.[31] Others have achieved similar feats, such as drought-resistant wheat, that should help if water shortages become more serious because of either population growth or environmental problems.[32]

Even technology companies are getting excited about resource management. Both IBM and Intel have joined a working group to study how information and technology can be used to improve water management in an effort to minimize waste. Cnet News green tech reporter Martin LaMonica notes that "water systems even in developed countries like the U.S. are notoriously outdated, with faulty pipes—some of them still made of wood—resulting in 25 percent to 45 percent lost water."[33] Yet even if resources can be properly managed, the issue of pollution is still a big concern.

OLDER, RICHER, AND CLEANER

Like longevity, eco-action is correlated with wealth. Numerous studies have shown that as people get richer, they turn more of their attention to making their environment cleaner. Peter Huber, a scholar at the New York–based Manhattan Institute, puts it this way: "It is wealth that gives ordinary families the confidence to be generous to the world beyond. It is the rich who can be thin because they know they will always have plenty to eat. It is the rich who can cherish the wilderness because they no longer have to choose between their own survival and nature's."[34]

Such an argument builds on the idea that every individual has certain needs, such as nourishment and clothing, that must be met before she or he can begin to care about the health of the trees or rivers. Psychologist Abraham Maslow's hierarchy of needs is often used as a way to think more clearly about how this works. Figure 3.3 shows the Maslow pyramid outlining human needs, starting with the most basic.

As individuals move up the various levels in the pyramid, their motivation to be active in better managing issues like air pollution and waste tends to rise. For instance, University of Chicago economist Don Coursey found that income levels are strongly correlated with concern about the environment. Income, of course, is instrumental in ensuring food, water, and safety, and a fulfilling career con-

FIGURE 3.3

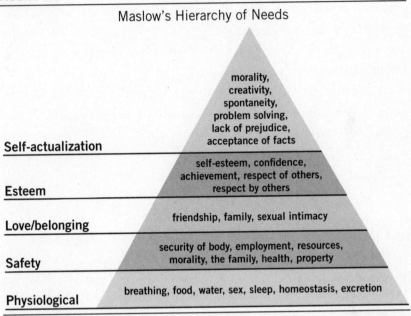

Maslow's Hierarchy of Needs

Self-actualization — morality, creativity, spontaneity, problem solving, lack of prejudice, acceptance of facts

Esteem — self-esteem, confidence, achievement, respect of others, respect by others

Love/belonging — friendship, family, sexual intimacy

Safety — security of body, employment, resources, morality, the family, health, property

Physiological — breathing, food, water, sex, sleep, homeostasis, excretion

Source: Based on A. H. Maslow, "A Theory of Human Motivation," *Psychological Review* 50 (1943): 370–396.

tributes to personal well-being. Unsurprisingly, then, Coursey found that when income increases, concern for the environment does, too, leading him to conclude that the demand for environmental quality is "similar to the demand for new cars and private education."[35]

Princeton economists Gene Grossman and Alan Krueger made a similar argument and were among the first to demonstrate how this works in a 1991 paper about free trade.[36] They showed that, although "economic growth brings an initial phase of deterioration" in environmental quality, it is "followed by a subsequent phase of improvement."[37] Such an inverted U curve is often referred to as an environmental Kuznets curve (EKC), named after economist Simon Kuznets, who argued that as incomes rise, there is an initial phase of great inequality, which is followed later by a reduction of that inequality. This theory, which won Kuznets the Nobel Prize in 1971, works in a similar way when applied to the environment. A typical EKC looks like Figure 3.4,

FIGURE 3.4

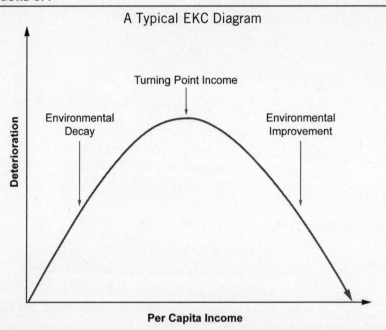

A Typical EKC Diagram

SOURCE: Based on Bruce Yandle, Madhusudan Bhattarai, and Maya Vijayaraghavan, "Environmental Kuznets Curves: A Review of Findings, Methods, and Policy Implications," Research Study 02-1 (Bozeman, MT: PERC, April 2004), www.perc.org/pdf/rs02_1a.pdf.

and the actual numbers will vary depending on the environmental problems described (air pollutants, deforestation, etc.).

As the figure indicates, once people hit a certain level of wealth (the "turning point income"), they begin to take better care of the environment. This happens because the individuals involved finally reach a point where they can afford to pay attention to environmental problems. As Maslow's pyramid helps to explain, people tend to focus on the most obvious and pressing concerns first, such as cleaning up roads and waterways, and then later on other higher-level problems, such as air particulates and deforestation.

This pattern has occurred, and continues to occur, in developed countries like the United States and is now beginning in developing countries. According to Grossman and Krueger, the general tipping point at which individuals are secure enough to focus more on the environment is a per capita income of $8,000. Other scholars have come up with different estimates, but the argument is not over whether this phenomenon happens but at what income level it happens.[38] Of course, not all environmental problems are tackled at once, and even wealthy countries like the United States have still not addressed every single issue. For instance, carbon emissions continue to be an issue that persists in the United States, but recent studies show that the EKC turning point for this issue may kick in at a per capita income of $30,000.[39] Because personal per capita income in the United States was $38,615 in 2007, this may help to explain why the issue has been so often in the news and President Barack Obama's administration has been working so hard to create policies to fix the problem, including announcing a goal to reduce carbon emissions by more than 80 percent by the year 2050.[40] It may also partially explain why so many companies are jumping to do what they can to help the environment. For instance, in the last few years Microsoft and Google have subsidized employee purchases of hybrid cars, Sprint released a cell phone called "Reclaim" made of 80 percent recycled materials, and Wal-Mart started a "Personal Sustainability Project" whereby employees voluntarily adopted "habits that positively impact the environment."

This discussion about the link between wealth and concern for the environment is not meant to imply that people in poorer countries don't care about the environment, but it does mean that the rich are in a better position to *do* something about it. Add to this reality a longer life span and the increased experience that goes with it, and the argument that people will continue to get greener as their health spans grow becomes even stronger. That's because the longer someone will be around, the more likely he is to think about his needs in the longer term.

It wouldn't make sense, for instance, to implement policies that will result in pollution fifty years from now if the people making those very policies will personally have to deal with the results in fifty years.

As Carl Safina, environmentalist and cofounder of the Blue Ocean Institute, puts it, "Conservation is not a trade-off between the economy and the environment. It is a trade-off between the short and long term."[41]

Indeed, as life expectancies have been rising, so have our concerns and efforts toward preserving the environment, particularly in those democratic countries where market competition drives companies to be good corporate citizens and the will of the people pushes government to set higher and higher standards for businesses. President Bill Clinton, closely attuned to the issues of the day, said in 2000, "From our inner cities to our pristine wild lands, we have worked hard to ensure that every American has a clean and healthy environment. We've rid hundreds of neighborhoods of toxic waste dumps, and taken the most dramatic steps in a generation to clean the air we breathe. We have made record investments in science and technology to protect future generations from the threat of global warming."[42]

Political statements such as this help to show how those leading democratic institutions can and do aid in the goal of cleaner environments, which backs up numerous studies that demonstrate a strong linkage among political power, civil rights, property rights, and a better environment (see Figure 3.5).[43] Because cleaner environments are intrinsically linked with longer life expectancies, there is an important feedback loop among these three items: empowering political institutions (democracy and property rights), a clean environment, and health (which produces economic growth).

The reality that a strong economy, healthy political institutions, and longer life expectancies support the environment can also be demonstrated through seemingly ordinary examples, such as how a community's trash is managed. For instance, in 2009 The Economist released a special report on waste management showing stark contrasts between rich and poor countries and, by association, high-life-expectancy countries and low-life-expectancy countries.

It is true that richer and longer-lived countries generate more waste per person. This only makes sense: if someone can afford to

FIGURE 3.5

Linkages Among Political Institutions, Health, and the Environment

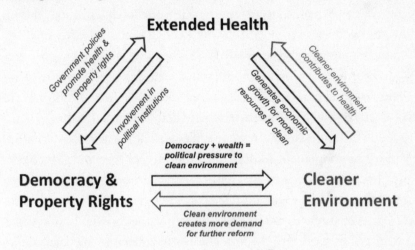

buy more items over a longer period of time, she will have more garbage to throw away. It is also true that in poorer countries the personal motivation to recycle is much higher because recycling is cheaper than purchasing new items. But even with these realities, the richer, longer-lived countries do a better job at managing waste and making sure it doesn't harm the environment.

Consider the difference between a landfill in India, where people have a per capita income of $950 and a life expectancy of sixty-three years, and one in the United Kingdom, where people have a per capita income of $42,740 and a life expectancy of seventy-nine years.[44] Both landfills are the same size, yet the one in India takes in almost twice as much waste per year and is much more toxic.

The Indian landfill, called Deonar dumping ground, takes all types of waste and "has no budget for fencing or crowd control, let alone modern environmental safeguards."[45] At their peril, locals comb through the garbage. "Leachate," a fancy name for rainwater that trickles through the landfill picking up toxins and pollutants, seeps into the local creeks and then into the Arabian Sea. According to

The Economist's report, no one knows how dangerous the Deonar leachate is because the water is not tested. And the situation only gets worse because there is no system to collect the landfill gas and "during the dry season several fires break out every day and smolder away, releasing plumes of acrid smoke."

In contrast, the British landfill, called Pitsea, is located on the banks of the River Thames near London, and can accept only municipal and commercial solid waste because mixing liquid and solid wastes, or hazardous and nonhazardous wastes, is illegal. The owner of the landfill, Veolia Environnement Group, must follow very specific rules to prevent leachate by constructing barriers and then treating any contaminated water before it can be released. Strict standards of testing exist for levels of contaminants such as ammonia, heavy metals, and other chemicals. In addition, "the firm also has to collect the methane emitted by the landfill, which has meant sinking 1000 wells at regular intervals across the 120 hectare site."[46] Access to the site is controlled, as are the air quality, dust, and odors. And in what is perhaps a sign that regulators are already thinking about their rapidly extending health spans, "Veolia must set aside money to ensure that the leachate continues to be treated, the gas collected, the local environment monitored and any damage remedied after the landfill stops accepting waste, which is meant to happen in 2015."[47] Add to this the fact that the firm's liability "lasts as long as the landfill continues to generate leachate or gas," which could be practically forever, and we can see that the wealthier and longer-lived country is thinking very long term.[48]

NEXT STEPS

There are new technologies on the horizon that promise to make the planet a cleaner and healthier place. For instance, it looks increasingly likely that societies will be able to turn more of their waste into fertilizer or energy.[49] Such processes, if they were to become common, would revolutionize the way we think about garbage, perhaps even creating new and vibrant competition to collect trash.

How could waste be turned into fuel? One method involves a field known as synthetic biology, in which engineering principles are applied to biological systems. Using DNA sequencing and synthesis, scientists can re-engineer organisms like bacteria, yeast, and algae, thereby creating mini chemical factories that can turn all sorts of waste, including paper waste and carbon dioxide, into fuel. One engineer working on such methods is Dr. Jay Keasling, a professor of chemical engineering at the University of California, Berkeley and CEO of one of the government's Joint BioEnergy Institutes established to find alternatives to foreign oil.

Before training his sights on fuel, Dr. Keasling engineered a new microorganism by inserting wormwood genes into a yeast cell. The resulting, incredibly important microbe could turn sugar into artemisinin, a powerful antimalaria drug. Making artemisinin used to be a slow and expensive process, but now the drug can be made more quickly and for pennies per dose. Malaria kills more than 1 million people every year, so Dr. Keasling's invention, funded by the Bill and Melinda Gates Foundation, will make a huge difference, particularly in poorer regions of the world where malaria is more common. This feat earned Dr. Keasling the honors of being selected as *Discover* magazine's "scientist of the year" in 2006 and being awarded the first annual Biotech Humanitarian Award by the Biotechnology Industry Organization in 2009.[50] Yet how does an engineer go from making an antimalaria drug to helping produce fuel for cars and jets?

In an interview on a popular television program, Keasling explained that the drug his microorganisms create "is a hydrocarbon, much like the gas you put in your automobile."[51] It doesn't take much imagination to see why the U.S. Department of Energy picked him to lead one of its $134 million initiatives to create environmentally friendly biofuels. And Dr. Keasling is not the only one working on using synthetic biology to create cleaner fuel.

Another heavy hitter in this space is Dr. J. Craig Venter, the scientist mentioned in Chapter 2 who is known for sequencing the human genome. Dr. Venter's for-profit company, Synthetic Genomics, aims to "engineer superior strains of algae, and to define and develop the best systems for large-scale cultivation of algae and conversion of their products into useful biofuels."[52] To this end, in July 2009 the company landed a $600 million deal with ExxonMobil, the largest publicly traded international oil and gas company, an important sign that the field is looking promising.

"Algae is the ultimate biological system using sunlight to capture and convert carbon dioxide into fuel," Dr. Venter said.[53] Using CO_2 as a raw material would convert waste into energy and help fight global warming at the same time. ExxonMobil's money will go toward long-term research and development exploring the most efficient and cost-effective organisms and methods to produce next-generation algal biofuel. Generating fuel this way will certainly help limit CO_2 pollution and may be in use sooner than most of us expect.

For instance, commercial airlines have already flown a number of successful test flights using various biofuel–jet fuel blends. According to Boeing, these included a "Virgin Atlantic flight using a coconut- and babassu-derived biofuel blend; an Air New Zealand flight using a jatropha-derived biofuel blend; a Continental Airlines flight using a blend of algae- and jatropha-derived biofuel; and a Japan Airlines flight using an algae-, jatropha- and camelina-derived biofuel blend."[54] Using just 50 percent biofuel during a twelve-hour flight would save 1.43 metric tons of fuel and reduce carbon dioxide emissions by about 4.5 metric tons, making the technology a step in the right direction.

Aside from synthetic biology, there are other technologies that also aim to help solve carbon emissions problems created by burning fossil fuels for energy. The possibilities include (but are certainly not limited to) producing energy from advanced nanotech solar panels and generating power from the once disgraced area known as "cold fusion."

Back in 1989 scientists Stanley Pons and Martin Fleischmann announced they had discovered cold fusion, or a nuclear reaction that happens at a slower rate than hot fusion, without the dangerous radiation. A media frenzy followed over expectations of this clean and cheap energy source, but the excitement quickly dissipated when other researchers had trouble replicating Pons and Fleischmann's work. Despite this disappointment, top scientists continued to investigate cold fusion possibilities because, if perfected, the reward would be a seemingly never-ending clean energy source that would generate more energy than was used to create it. Now, it appears that some scientists have made progress. In April 2009, *60 Minutes* televised a story about researchers who are getting closer to figuring out how to turn the idea into a reliable energy source. "The potential is for an energy source that would run your car for three, four years, for example. And you'd take it in for service every four years and they'd give you a new power supply," Dr. Michael McKubre of SRI International labs told the *60 Minutes* crew.[55]

Such statements might sound fantastical, yet representatives from the U.S. Navy have publicly said that cold fusion is possible, and a number of top scientists are currently working on techniques to make it a more stable and reliable energy source.[56] The main issue with cold fusion, it seems, is that the elements involved are unstable, resulting in different levels of energy being released in each experiment even though the experiment is apparently being done in the same manner each time. Such quandaries are, of course, what makes science interesting to scientists, and at some point one of them will figure out what is going on so that this energy source can be properly harnessed. In the meantime, nanotechnology looks well poised to help solar energy become more efficient.

Nanotechnology is the science of the very small. A manipulation of matter at the level of tiny individual atoms and molecules, nanotechnology is an information technology because, as futurist and inventor Ray Kurzweil says, it is the business of "applying information processes to create intricate new devices at the molecular level."[57] Because these technologies tend to progress exponentially, he predicts that solar power will scale up to produce *all* the energy needs of the earth's people in twenty years. He often reminds audiences that "there is 10,000 times more sunlight than we need to meet 100 percent of our energy needs, and the technology needed for collecting and storing it is about to emerge as the field of solar energy is going to advance exponentially in accordance with the Law of Accelerating Returns. That law yields a doubling of price performance in information technologies every year."[58] Whether or not we believe Kurzweil's projections, it is true that nano-engineered fuel cells already exist and solar panels are continually becoming smaller and more efficient. For instance, a company called Nanosolar has developed technology that enables the production of one-hundred-times-thinner solar cells, with much greater efficiency.

Apart from driving a revolution in solar technologies, nanotechnology is poised to help in such areas as agriculture, defense, environmental improvement, transport, consumer products, and health-extending medicine.[59] Already used to build stronger, lighter materials for baseball bats and tennis rackets, nanotech will certainly be used in the future for lighter, fuel-efficient vehicles. It has also shown great promise for cleaning both water and environmental spills, such as oil in the sea. In 2008 MIT researchers announced that they had created a mesh of nanowires that could soak up as much as twenty times its weight in oil and could be recycled many times over.[60] Such a tool could help with any future catastrophes along the lines of the Deepwater Horizon oil spill in the Gulf of Mexico, as well as other smaller spills that are already endangering the oceans. The team created a prototype of its autonomous water-cleaning robot, SeaSwarm, and successfully tested it in August 2010.[61]

Yet despite such benefits, some individuals and groups are concerned that nanotechnology could have unintended environmental consequences that may make us think twice about going forward. Just like coal blackened the skies when humans first started burning it, there are concerns that the earth could become littered with nano-dust. Some even see a day when tiny and intelligent nano robots, or "nano-bots," would be able to self-replicate and pose a danger to all life on earth. This leads us then to an important question: is nanotech the coal of the second industrial revolution, and could its use lead to greater destruction than we have ever seen before?

PRECAUTIONARY PRINCIPLE VERSUS INNOVATION

Perhaps the most famous critic of nanotechnology is Bill Joy, a co-founder and former chief scientist of Sun Microsystems. In a *Wired* magazine article in 2000, Joy worried that "we are being propelled into a new century with no plan, no control, no brakes." Specifically, he worried about robots, engineered organisms, and nano-bots that can self-replicate. "A bomb is blown up only once," he wrote, "but one bot can become many, and quickly get out of control."[62] Such a scenario was scary enough for fiction writer Michael Crichton to seize upon as the main theme for his 2002 book *Prey*, in which a cloud of predator-programmed nano-bots escape from the lab where they were made. When television interviewer Charlie Rose asked Crichton why he chose self-replicating technology as his subject, Crichton replied that he wanted to write about the "Frankenstein" of today. "The monster of today would look very different," he said.[63]

Yet self-replicating nanotechnology is not likely to be created anytime soon, and making decisions based on scenarios such as Crichton's *Prey* would be foolish. Nevertheless, radical environmentalists such as Bill McKibben argue that because new technologies could get out of our control, we should stop pursuing them.[64]

But banning technology doesn't usually work as a safety mechanism. Instead, government bans tend to send the targeted activity underground, where only people with malicious intentions will use it. Likewise, banning nanotechnology would also mean giving up its benefits, many of which have nothing to do with self-replicating machines. Useful nanotech already exists that is non-self-replicating, and the fear of self-replicating machines is theoretical and based on assumptions about a technology that doesn't yet exist.[65] Of course, that doesn't mean that scientists shouldn't be thinking about how to avoid such problems. That the concern has been expressed so far in advance of a possible threat means that if it ever comes to pass, scientists will be in a better position to disable it. Indeed, respected groups such as the Foresight Institute exist to bring together experts to discuss such scenarios, as well as other potential problems, in order to ensure the beneficial implementation of nanotechnology. Christine Peterson, president of Foresight, says that out-of-control nanobots are an unlikely outcome of the advancement of nanotechnology "because we can gain the benefits of molecular manufacturing without making any systems able to self-replicate. It's not necessary, and it's hard to do, so it seems unlikely."[66] Instead, she says, there are other, more realistic concerns, such as nanoparticle toxicity and potential nanotech-related arms races, that the public and experts in the field need to consider. This leads us back to the question of whether nanotechnology will be to the second industrial revolution what coal was to the first. Some groups fear this is the case.

For instance, the Canadian-based ETC Group has called for greater government oversight of already-existing nanotechnology products, such as the small particles used to make sunscreen clear (as opposed to white) and the small silver particles used in washing machines to better clean clothes. "Nanotechnology—including nanobiotechnology—has been pegged by industry and governments to become the world's largest and fastest industrial revolution—dwarfing history's past technological upheavals," the group wrote in a pamphlet. "Given the concerns raised over nanoparticle contamination in living organisms, Heads of State attending the World Summit on Sustainable Development should declare an immediate moratorium on commercial production of new nanomaterials and launch a transparent global process for evaluating the socio-economic, health and environmental implications of the technology."[67]

Such concerns are not surprising. History shows that when new technology makes humans better off, sometimes temporary problems are created. With burning coal, this meant that people put up with polluted skies in exchange for a reliable source of heat and cooking fuel until there were enough pressure and incentive to find cleaner, better ways to produce energy to maintain standards of living and ultimately live longer. Is the same thing happening when it comes to nanotechnology?

So far, the evidence doesn't point that way. Sometimes technology just makes humans better off, period. What is encouraging, however, is that there are a number of watchdog groups aiming to make sure we avoid waiting too long before we fix any problems that might crop up. For instance, Andrew Maynard of the Environmental Working Group coauthored an important paper showing that direct inhalation of carbon nanotubes "may lead to mesothelioma, cancer of the lining of the lungs caused by exposure to asbestos."[68] Of course, using a sunscreen with nanotech or an iPod made from nanomaterials does not pose such risks because consumers will not be inhaling them, but the study does point to potential risks for workers in factories using nanotechnology.

In addition to watchdog groups looking for potential problems with nanoparticles, various groups aim to establish a set of best practices for developing and testing the technology. That was certainly not a luxury that the people of the first industrial revolution could claim and goes to show how the societal mind-set and circumstances have changed with increased wealth.

One suggestion for moving forward safely was advanced in a paper released by the Environmental Defense Fund in partnership with DuPont. In June 2005 they created an initiative called the Nano Risk Framework. Writing in the *Wall Street Journal*, the leaders of the two organizations said they were hoping to make nanotechnology as safe as possible.

"An early and open examination of the potential risks of a new product or technology is not just good common sense—it's good business strategy. We need to make sure this assessment takes place now for today's 'next big thing'—nanotechnology," said Fred Krupp, president of the Environmental Defense Fund, and Chad Holliday, chairman and CEO of DuPont.[69] In 2007 the groups published the results of their work. They recommended six steps to evaluate the safety of nanomaterials: describing the materials and applications; profiling life cycles; evaluating risks; assessing risk management techniques; deciding, documenting, and acting; and reviewing and adapting.[70] Essentially, the

plan comprises examining the facts, implementing fixes where necessary, and continuing to monitor the situation.

This type of strategy is a good middle ground between being
overly cautious and not monitoring the technology at all. Some activists, however, have rejected such reasonable methods of action,
instead preferring to invoke an idea called the "precautionary principle," which essentially states that unless industry can prove with 100
percent certainty that a product is safe, then it can't be produced or
sold. This principle might sound good in theory, but it can never be
fulfilled because there are many variables involved with product
safety and problems often don't present themselves in obvious ways.

Not long after the Environmental Defense Fund and DuPont released their reasonable guidelines, Greenpeace, the American Federation of Labor–Congress of Industrial Organizations, and a number
of affiliated groups released a statement calling for a "precautionary
foundation: product manufacturers and distributors must bear the
burden of proof to demonstrate the safety of their products." The
statement argued that "lack of data or evidence of specific harm cannot substitute for a reasonable certainty of safety."[71]

Such a reaction is overkill, and the burden it would impose on innovation would seriously threaten the future of technology development. Indeed, even proregulation observers of nanotechnology, such
as the Center for Responsible Nanotechnology (CRN), recognize that
such a strict regime would be harmful. If the precautionary principle
leads to innovation being squashed, or to "inaction," Chris Phoenix
and Mike Treder of CRN argue, the risks "may be greater than the
risks of action."[72] Another way to put it is that a fear of risk could lead
to irrational delays that would then deprive humanity of great benefits, such as a cleaner environment and increased health spans. Perhaps inventor Ray Kurzweil said it best when he argued, "We need
to better balance the risks of new technology against the known harm
of delay."[73]

There are important and legitimate questions about the effect of
greater health spans on population growth, resource availability, and

health of the environment. Even though the well-known Malthusian story line maintains that the only thing about population that matters is the numbers, as this chapter showed, it is not just a numbers game. The effects of population growth also depend on human *action*, which tends to get more creative as prices rise or shortages become imminent. It is true that innovations in technology that ultimately lead to cleaner environments and longer health spans can sometimes have unintended consequences. Progress is never perfect, and there can be snags along the way. However, in looking at the trends, we can see that even when there are downsides to a particular wealth- or health-enhancing technology, the problem is often fixed once the population reaches a point where it feels secure in spending the resources to do so. Likewise, as people live longer, they are not only likely to become "greener" in their thinking, but they will also have a richer experience to draw on when deciding how to best care for the environment.

But just because Mother Nature can handle longer-lived people doesn't automatically mean that she should. Next, we will turn our attention to the central moral and philosophical questions surrounding health extension.

CHAPTER 4

The Longevity Divide

Does Living Longer Mean Living Better?

IN JANUARY 2002 the President's Council on Bioethics was asked by its chairman, Dr. Leon Kass, to read and discuss "The Birthmark," a short story by nineteenth-century American author Nathaniel Hawthorne. Odd as it might be for a U.S. public policy deliberation on stem cells to consider a fictional work, Dr. Kass's message became clear.

Hawthorne's story is about a scientist who marries a beautiful woman whose only imperfection is a small birthmark on her face. In an effort to erase the mark, the scientist winds up accidentally killing his wife. The tale is meant to warn humanity of the evils of scientific hubris. As we shall see, this is not the first time Dr. Kass used fictional works to make a point about reality—a strategy questioned by many. In response, Pulitzer Prize–winning journalist Ellen Goodman asked who, if anyone, was "ready to argue that Alzheimer's disease should be protected from the mad hand of a scientist?"[1] So whereas some see scientific advances as a movement toward "perfectionism," others see them as responsible action directed toward reducing human suffering.

Although life extension is not about chasing perfection per se, it is about making humans healthier for longer periods of time, an idea that some reject on moral grounds. This chapter will consider the key philosophical objections to extending human life expectancy, such as the idea that superlongevity is unnatural and driven by hubris. Or to put the issue in more general terms, is it a good thing to attempt to slow down the aging process and extend healthy human life?

NATURE AND HUMANITY

Today, a plethora of food and cosmetic companies market their products with "natural" labels, usually meaning that they are not filled with synthetic chemicals and other artificial ingredients that may be detrimental to our health. Even though positive in that context, "natural" isn't automatically good. For instance, it is natural for teeth to rot, but we have found ways to protect ourselves from that rather nasty problem. It is also natural for volcanoes to erupt, earthquakes to occur, and polar bears to rip apart humans who enter their habitat. Indeed, since the beginning of time humans have been devising ways to escape the problems of nature. Philosopher Thomas Hobbes had it right in the seventeenth century when he famously described the human condition as one of "continual fear, and danger of violent death; and the life of man, solitary, poor, nasty, brutish and short." In other words, until men and women started finding ways to overcome the state of nature, life certainly wasn't rosy.

In the twenty-first century, life is better than it was in the world of Hobbes. Consider that as recently as 1850 life expectancy was only forty-three years, the air was visibly polluted, refrigeration wasn't widely available for fresh food, central heating didn't exist, the chances of getting an infection from unhygienic water or streets was extremely high, and vaccines against many diseases such as rubella and polio weren't invented yet. Fortunately, ensuring our safety has become easier, and humans now enjoy longer and healthier lives. Despite this success, some scholars and activists argue that healthy life extension shouldn't be taken any further. Most noted of these is Dr. Kass, who was President George W. Bush's appointee as chairman of the President's Council on Bioethics from 2001 to 2005. Dr. Kass is squarely in the anti-life-extension camp, arguing that using technology to extend healthy life is "incompatible" with human nature.[2] His point of view may seem strange, if not outright Luddite, but many share this perspective, so it is worth attempting to understand the rationale behind it.

"This is a question in which our very humanity is at stake," Kass writes, "not only in the consequences, but also in the very meaning of the choice. For to argue that human life would be better without death is, I submit, to argue that human life would be better being something other than human."[3] Although some people might be tempted to dismiss this opinion as the musings of a right-wing pundit, similar arguments are also made by some on the left. For instance, Bill McKibben, a well-known author and left-leaning environmentalist, strongly opposes "techno-longevity." He explains that, "like everything before us, we will rot our way back into the woof and warp of the planet. That's what humans are: animals that can anticipate their demise. And being human has always meant being, in some irreducible way, yourself. Not a genetically programmed machine designed for maximum performance."[4] Someday, he says, death "will happen." "But I'll take it. I can deal with being a real human."[5]

Even if such statements appeal to our love of nature, it's not true that technology use is antihuman. Humans have a long history of creating tools and technologies to improve health and lengthen lives. Humans are still human even after having their eyes fixed with laser surgery, terrible diseases prevented with vaccines, and cancer sometimes beat with surgery and other techniques. As bioethicist Arthur Caplan points out, "We don't think of ourselves as being engineered for improvement, but we are. We are travelling, eating, flying, computing, and perceiving in ways that are distinct improvements upon what would be possible using only our natural endowments."[6] Indeed, human nature includes the capacity not only to survive, but also to survive longer and better if possible. Despite such an obvious point, Kass, McKibben, and others persist in claiming that advancements leading to longer lives will lead to a "less human" future. Let's examine some of the more detailed arguments for this proposition.

From Kass's perspective, the reasons to stop fighting aging touch on at least three things he associates with human nature. First, if people were to live longer, they would lose what he calls "interest and engagement." What would a person do, he asks, after having been "CEO of Microsoft, a member of Congress, or the President of Harvard for a quarter of a century?"[7] Kass's point is not just a worry about boredom but also a real concern about purpose. Such a question reveals pessimism about the creativity and adaptability of humans, which ironically make up part of the human nature Kass seeks to protect. In viewing the world as it is now, in which greater life expectancies have already allowed individuals to live long enough to reinvent themselves after being a CEO or even president of the United States, his question is easily answered.

What is Bill Gates doing now that he has finished being CEO of Microsoft? He has dedicated his life to improving the world for others through the Bill and Melinda Gates Foundation. He is a brilliant individual, and the world is fortunate to have him still playing an active part. Not only has he been instrumental in directing researchers to find a way to beat malaria, but he is also thinking hard about how to solve the world's energy problems. Similarly, Jimmy Carter, Bill Clinton, and George W. Bush have all been active trying to help solve the world's problems long after holding the top political job in the United States. For example, the Clinton Bush Haiti Fund, in which the two former presidents joined together, raises money to help earthquake survivors in Haiti.[8]

Dr. Kass's second concern with longer life expectancy is what he calls a deficit in "seriousness and aspiration." He worries that if immortality is one day possible, life won't carry the same meaning because there will be so much of it. He argues that "mortality makes life matter."[9] Kass is certainly not the only person to reach this conclusion—it is a common refrain of antilongevity activists. For instance, Daniel Callahan, codirector of the Yale-Hastings Program in Ethics and Health Policy and president emeritus of the Hastings Center, has written that "more life beyond a certain point seems to offer no proportionate gains" and that people in developed countries "already live long enough to accomplish most reasonable human ends."[10] Many readers will disagree with this assertion because time is often in short supply, but the question is, why do some scholars assume that life is valuable only if it is restricted?

To better explain his assertion, Kass points to mythology, where immortal gods such as Zeus and Athena "live shallow and rather frivolous lives."[11] But extrapolating from fictional works is not the best way to reason about the future. People can be shallow and frivolous independent of their longevity, and we should remember that fictional works written at times when there was no real prospect of extending lives greatly are likely to reflect sour grapes and a rationalizing of aging and death. But perhaps more importantly, immortality defined as living forever no matter what is implausible.[12] As University of Manchester bioethics professor John Harris puts it, "Immortality is not invulnerability."[13] Even if human beings can be repaired indefinitely, accidents will still happen and new diseases will arise. In short, life will never be certain. And in this book we are not considering the consequences of immortality; we are looking at the effects of what some view as radical longevity—a doubling of healthy life expectancy to around 150 years.

Finally, Kass's third antilongevity argument is his belief that death promotes "virtue and moral excellence." Without impending death, he concludes, it is not possible to be noble because nobility requires "spending the precious coinage of the time of our lives."[14] Again, this argument hinges on the idea of scarcity, but it turns out to be a red herring because repair of bodies does not guarantee invulnerability. And in any case, the moral value of a good deed does not depend on the death of the person performing the deed. Fighting for freedom is noble in and of itself, and death in the line of fire is a tragedy. Likewise, there are many noble causes that aren't usually correlated with the death of the people involved in them, such as finding cures to diseases that cause human suffering or helping children out of poverty.

Arguments against life extension are often simply an appeal to the status quo. They are efforts to instill worry that if humans were to live longer, the world in some way would not be right—it wouldn't be noble, beautiful, or exciting. But what is noble, beautiful, and exciting about withholding efforts at ameliorating human suffering? The answer is nothing. Instead, a better argument, made by Harris and others, is that there is a moral obligation to help humans live longer, healthier lives because *everything* individuals have is based on life. As Harris writes, "To decide to withhold a benefit is in a sense to harm the individual we decline to benefit."[15] That is, if we have the ability to help others avoid death for longer than they otherwise would, not pursuing that goal is tantamount to murder. Some may say this reasoning goes too far, but it is certainly morally wrong to work against making people healthier. Nevertheless, all potential ethical issues arising from significant life extension should be considered. One concern that often comes up is that lengthening human life expectancy is too dangerous.

THE PRUDENCE OF AUGMENTING NATURE

As we learned in Chapter 1, humans have often imagined that in trying to extend their health spans, they may accidentally cause something terrible to happen. Dr. Frankenstein's monster is a literary example of that fear—in trying to re-create life, the well-intentioned doctor instead creates a monster. In small doses, fear of mistakes is useful because it reminds us to be careful. In larger doses, this fear can halt progress altogether. We often declare, in one context or another, that we "should not play God," but perhaps a better way to frame the issue here is to ask if attempting to augment nature is prudent.

It's true that humans often make mistakes when attempting to fix things. There are many examples, particularly when it comes to tackling complex scientific, technological, or ecological problems. Australian philosopher C. A. J. Coady points out that his country is suffering from the negative effects of the well-intentioned importation from Hawaii of cane toads to control sugar cane pests. "Adult animals have few natural predators so their population has exploded throughout north and central Australia, and threatens regions further south," he explains. "They have high toxicity and are fatally poisonous if eaten by most native animals and they are capable of eating small native toads and native frogs."[16] This disaster, Coady reports, has led some to conclude that "it's pretty dangerous to play God, especially with complex eco-systems." A similar case, he notes, is often made by those worried about what will happen when we further tinker with human genes. For instance, William Hurlbut, a Stanford-based physician who served on George W. Bush's bioethics council, warns that "genetics is very complicated; most genes affect many traits and most traits are affected by many genes."[17]

Those who worry about genetic experiments have cautionary examples at their disposal. For example, in 1999 eighteen-year-old Jesse Gelsinger died after an experimental genetic therapy caused his liver disease to spiral out of control. Then, in 2002 French researchers used gene therapy to cure two patients with "bubble boy disease," but the unfortunate side effect appeared to be leukemia.[18] These examples prompted technologist and author Ramez Naam to note that "gene therapy has had a tough decade, because of poor safety outcomes."[19] But gene therapy is not the only useful advance to hit rough spots in its infancy. Many therapies with great potential experienced problems when first developed. For example, although vaccines have saved millions of lives from the pain of whooping cough or the iron lung needed for polio victims, their use was not always smooth sailing. Ann Arbor medical professors Alexandra Minna Stern and Howard Markel remind us that "the optimism about the polio vaccine in spring 1955 was temporarily muted after 200 children contracted disease (fatal for five children) from a vaccine containing active wild-type polio virus that was manufactured by Cutter Laboratories in California."[20] Fortunately, vaccines have become much safer and the news about genetic engineering is getting better as well.

Despite past problems with gene therapy, new discoveries allow for hope. For instance, Pfizer's drug Crizotinib, which inhibits a genetic

mutation in lung cancer cells, shrunk or stabilized tumors in around
90 percent of the patients who took it.[21] There are also successful gene
therapy trials that have dramatically improved the vision of individuals, like nine-year-old Corey Haas (discussed in Chapter 2). Corey's
leber congenital amaurosis was completely cured with gene therapy at
the Children's Hospital of Philadelphia.[22] As of this writing, all of the
human patients who underwent the same gene therapy as Corey had
improved vision and none suffered from safety issues, perhaps marking
a turning point for the field.

Over time gene therapy and other methods of health enhancement will become clearer and safer. It would be a shame if researchers
were to stop investigating this important field because previous mistakes were made. But when it comes to augmenting nature, it is not
the doctors that some fear; it is the politicians.

THREAT OF EUGENICS?

It is one thing to augment nature in order to cure diseases and extend
life expectancy, but the same technologies that can be used for
health might also someday be used for political purposes. The idea of
state-sponsored eugenics spurs recollections of the Nazis' race-based
horrors and forced sterilization of the disabled in the United States
and other countries. In these cases, the evils carried out occurred because governments and their armies made it happen. Those who are
opposed to augmenting nature today, such as C. Ben Mitchell and
C. Christopher Hook, fellows at the Institute of Biotechnology and
the Human Future, make the argument that all genetic enhancements, from those of the Nazi regime to the genetic enhancements of
today, can be considered eugenics.[23]

Putting the Holocaust and longevity enhancements in the same
category doesn't make sense, however. Such a sweeping argument ignores the key difference between the two: longevity enhancements
are freely chosen, whereas government-enforced eugenics is not. As
feisty UK journalist Johann Hari puts it, today's enhancements have

"nothing to do with the evil of Nazi eugenics, which was imposed by the state and concerned not with producing healthier babies but with deranged race-theories."[24] Indeed, if someone chooses to make changes to his or her body, that should be a right.

In an ironic turning of the tables, present-day opponents of enhancements want to use the power of government to force people into certain genetic categories. The authoritarianism that was once associated with racism and sterilization can now be associated with those propping up the status quo. As Naam remarks, "It's those who oppose individual and family genetic choice who have, in essence, decided that there's a certain 'correct' genetic heritage for humanity (the one we have today) and that the populace should not be allowed any choice in the matter."[25] But just because freely chosen enhancements are reasonable doesn't mean that government should get heavily involved with people's choices.

Reason magazine's Ronald Bailey is in favor of genetic enhancements, yet he warns that "given the sorry history of government sponsored eugenics, it is vital that control over genetic engineering never be given to any governmental authority."[26] Indeed, if government were to get in the business of funding enhancements, the state would necessarily have to begin picking and choosing which enhancements were the best because limited resources would mean that all of them couldn't be funded. This would essentially move society down the slippery slope toward political control of designing humans. Even strategies like distributing government vouchers to children, which would not be tied to a specific enhancement, would not likely prevent the problems associated with state involvement.

In the case of vouchers, parents would hold the ultimate power over whether to enhance their children and could even decide not to use the subsidy if they wished. But at what point would not enhancing a child be thought of as child abuse? If a parent had the option to use a taxpayer-sponsored therapy to make his or her child healthier but didn't, how long would it be before children's rights groups calling for mandatory enhancements would appear? Such groups would surely appeal to philosophers like Ronald Dworkin, who has written that "if playing God means struggling to improve our species, bringing into our conscious designs a resolution to improve what God deliberately or nature blindly has evolved over eons, then the first principle of ethical individualism *commands* that struggle" (my emphasis).[27] If these arguments were convincing to a large enough group of voters, government and its political masters would be back in the business of deciding how humans should be designed, a potentially dangerous situation, as history demonstrates.

Yet even if state intentions don't turn nefarious, philosophers such as Harvard's Michael Sandel maintain that "eugenic parenting is objectionable because it expresses and entrenches a certain stance toward the world—a stance of mastery and domination that fails to appreciate the gifted character of human powers and achievements, and misses the part of freedom that consists in a persisting negotiation with the given."[28] The words "gift" and "given" sound like yet another appeal to nature. It is no particular "gift" to die at 80 rather than at 150, so Dr. Sandel seems here to be appealing to the human sense of fear about change and attempting to showcase the status quo as a good in and of itself. But perhaps because that argument isn't completely convincing, Dr. Sandel offers a more practical one based on insurance fears.

Dr. Sandel suggests that if individuals were responsible for their own fortune, rather than at the mercy of nature, then healthier people would have a reduced incentive to help the unhealthy. He writes that "since people do not know whether or when various ills will befall them, they pool their risk by buying health insurance and life insurance." If, however, life-extension technologies advanced to the point that some were confident that they would live a long time, they would, Dr. Sandel argues, "opt out of the pool, causing other people's premiums to skyrocket. The solidarity of insurance would disappear as those with good genes fled the actuarial company of those with bad ones."[29]

This argument implies that the primary reason we feel the need to help others is that we selfishly worry that we will wind up like them. That may be one factor driving some people to help others, but to suggest it is the main reason is overly pessimistic and sounds more like a critique of the insurance business, which exists precisely because it charges people different rates based on their risks (think teenage drivers and car insurance). Indeed, Frances Kamm, one of Dr. Sandel's colleagues in Harvard's Philosophy Department, sees this flaw in his reasoning and urges him to "recall that Kant thought we had a duty to help people pursue even the ends they themselves had deliberately chosen because people matter in their own right."[30]

People do matter in their own right, which is why charity exists within communities and why developed nations send aid to less-developed ones. This brings up other important issues surrounding life extension, such as resource allocation and the potential for creating even larger divides between the wealthy and poor.

RESOURCE USE AND SOCIAL JUSTICE

Some scholars argue that time and money shouldn't be spent on new technologies because there are still so many people living in poverty. For instance, Dr. Audrey Chapman, a professor of community medicine and health care at the University of Connecticut Health Center, argues that "investing in new and very expensive high technologies for enhancement interventions while people in our own country lack access to basic health care and millions of people die prematurely of preventable diseases in poor countries would be yet another step toward moral bankruptcy."[31] Her argument is meant to play on "rich guilt," but it is nonsensical because it assumes an either/or choice and completely ignores the health benefits of new innovations that could potentially lift poorer communities faster than anything available now. Technology is spreading more quickly today than ever before, and even though it may not reach poor communities at the same time as wealthy ones, it will likely get to the former faster than past innovations did.

Nick Bostrom, professor of philosophy at the University of Oxford, helps to expose the weakness in Chapman's emotionally charged argument. He writes, "It is unclear why aging research should be singled out for blame or special concern in this regard. Many factors contribute to global inequality, and spending on gerontological research is such a minute fraction of the financial outlays of wealthy nations that it seems a bizarre place to look for savings to transfer to the poor."[32] Instead, he argues that using poverty as an excuse to not advance health care innovations is an irrational psychological reaction reminiscent of Stockholm syndrome, whereby hostages become emotionally attached to their captors. That is, just as kidnapping victims become advocates for their captors, individuals can become advocates for aging and death. He writes:

> Apologism for human senescence might be viewed as a psychological defense mechanism that many people deploy as a way of coping with their own inescapable "capture" by the aging process. But just as the emotional bonding observed in the Stockholm syndrome can become counterproductive when it leads hostages to actively assist their captors in thwarting rescue efforts by the police, so too our adaptive acceptance of aging may become a problem when it prevents us from implementing the most promising research programs for improving healthy life expectancy.[33]

To be clear, social justice does not require humanity to give up attempts to live healthier, longer, and more productive lives. In fact, the opposite is true. Because any good that humans can have or do in their lives depends on the fact that they *have* lives, it is of utmost importance that society work toward innovating in medical science. Fortunately, this is a goal that most humans instinctively pursue and support, despite the long list of antilongevity arguments covered in this chapter. At this point, it is worth recognizing another argument that fits in the Stockholm syndrome camp. It is the idea that life extension is not worth pursuing because it could allow bad people to live longer. Pulitzer Prize–winning science writer Jonathan Weiner puts the idea this way: "If biologists could have done for the dictators of the twentieth century what they can now do for roundworms and flies—double their life span—then Mao Zedong might still be alive. . . . Joseph Stalin would be alive, too, and perhaps going strong. You can argue that dictators seldom die of natural causes. But giving very bad men very long lives would not be good for the world."[34]

Implicit in Weiner's reasoning is the assumption that long life automatically translates into long reign as a dictator, but the two are not necessarily linked. In fact, the longer a dictator lives, the more likely it is that he will create enemies and increase his vulnerability to being ousted and brought to justice. That was the fate of Nazi war criminals who were still alive to receive judgment, and it would have been the fate of Chilean dictator Augusto Pinochet had he not suffered a heart attack and died before facing trial. Oddly, death has allowed many of humanity's biggest villains to escape answering for their behavior. In a longer-lived world, that wouldn't be the case, and if the threat of justice didn't mitigate their actions, at least society would be able to tip the scales in a more just direction. The argument that good people shouldn't get life extension because bad people will also get it is fatally flawed. By that logic, good people shouldn't get food or medicine either because bad people could also get it. Now, it is time to turn to issues of human rights.

HUMAN RIGHTS, GENETIC WARFARE, AND ECONOMIC DIVIDES

John Hopkins political scientist Francis Fukuyama argues that humans shouldn't meddle with their genetic code, even if it looks like the experiment will be safe and successful, because doing so could change politics in negative ways. Like Dr. Kass, Fukuyama fears that tinkering with human genes would lead to a significant change in human nature itself. He maintains that if technological enhancements changed human nature and not everyone were enhanced or if individuals were enhanced in different ways, then it would not be long before a serious case could be made that humans do not all deserve equal rights. As he puts it, "We do not want to disrupt either the unity or the continuity of human nature, and thereby the human rights that are based on it."[35]

This fear about rights is shared by those on both ends of the political spectrum. Whereas Fukuyama is an example from the right, Boston law professor George Annas is an example from the left. Annas is shriller than Fukuyama with his language and goes as far as to call genetic engineering "genocide." He says that it is a "crime against humanity" to "change the nature of what it means to be human, and to engage in species-altering activities."[36] Now, both authors also assume that enhancement could include other goals besides life extension, such as tweaks to boost intelligence or height, but engineering for longer life still falls under what they consider a change to human nature that could make humans less equal.

The conclusion that enhanced humans are not deserving of the same rights as nonenhanced humans (or vice versa) is reminiscent of the X-Men films, in which mutants who have superpowers are treated not as humans but as freaks in need of a cure. Such a scenario makes for an exciting movie, but in liberal democracies where equal political rights are well established, it's difficult to imagine that longevity enhancements would convince anyone to create unequal legal structures. But this begs the question, what makes us human?

It should go without saying that people are not all the same. Some have extensive intellectual abilities and talents, and others have few. Some are tall, and others are short. Some are blessed with genes that help to extend life, and others are not. Despite this acknowledged reality, Fukuyama argues that humans all share what he calls "Factor X," a "human essence." This essence is hard to define, he says, and can't be reduced to certain traits, but it includes an interaction of "moral choice, reason, language, sociability, sentience, emotions, and consciousness."[37] But both enhanced and unenhanced people would have these qualities, so this argument doesn't make much sense. Enhancement doesn't take anything away; it adds something. Attempting to define humanity in an abstract way simply leads to a squishy conversation that leaves little room for sensible discussions about the risks and benefits of enhancement.

The presumption that biological alterations for longevity will somehow cause individuals to become a different and scary species is not useful or convincing. For instance, if the gene that causes Huntington's disease could be removed, thereby allowing an individual to live longer, would that make her less human simply because she had been altered? Clearly, the answer would be no. What is the moral difference, then, between removing the Huntington's gene and tweaking a gene that might allow someone to live twice as long? It's a similar idea and wouldn't make the person any less human; it would simply fix something that caused the body to decay at a faster rate. It stands to reason that making humans healthier does not take anything away from their humanity. If Fukuyama and Annas have lost the debate here, they attempt to pick it back up by sounding alarms that serious political unrest could follow if some people were enhanced while others were not.

"If genetic engineering produces a different type of human, the relationship between these new humans and 'standard' humans is potentially, even likely, lethal," argues Annas. "Human history suggests differences will be socially magnified and that the two now different types of humans could consider each other as legitimate targets for preemptive extermination."[38]

Could warfare break out over life-extension technologies? It is true that technology is rarely adopted by everyone at the same time, and when life-extending science hits the market, it will almost certainly be used by the wealthy first. In the early stages of the technology's rollout, disparities in life expectancy between people within developed countries will surely grow, as will the difference in life expectancy between developed and developing countries. In light of this reality, it should be noted that rather shocking differences in life expectancy already exist, marking an unequal starting point in the first place.

According to 2010 estimates by the Central Intelligence Agency, the gap between the world's longest-lived country and shortest-lived country is a whopping 51 years—almost an entire lifetime (see Table 4.1). Angola, in south-central Africa, has the lowest life expectancy at 38.5 years, whereas Monaco, near southern France, has a life expectancy of 89.8 years. The United States ranks forty-ninth, with a life expectancy of 78.2 years.

Thus far, there have not been direct riots over life expectancy differences, although anger over economic divides may imply this possibility because health and wealth are tied together so closely. But divides are not only between nations; there are also significant divides within nations.

In the United States, when the most extreme cases are considered, there can be as much as a thirty-three-year gap in life expectancy between groups. For instance, a 2006 study by researchers at Harvard and the University of California, San Francisco found that Native American males in South Dakota had a life expectancy of fifty-eight years, compared with Asian American females in New Jersey, whose life expectancy was ninety-one years.[39] That's a huge divide. Scholars attempt to explain it on a number of levels, including community, race, education, health care access, and income. If advances in biotechnology wind up increasing this disparity by decades or more, this could become the biggest hot-button issue the country has ever faced.

Like Annas, Fukuyama thinks that differences in access to biotechnology could lead to outright war. He writes, "This is one of the few things in a politics of the future that people are likely to rouse themselves to fight over. By this I mean not just fighting metaphorically, in the sense of shouting matches among talking heads on TV and debates in Congress, but actually picking up guns and bombs and using them on other people."[40] Indeed, if some parts of the population are enjoying radically longer and healthier lives than others, life

TABLE 4.1

Top and Bottom Ten Countries Ranked for Life Expectancy, 2010

Top 10 Countries	2010 Life Expectancy Estimate
Monaco	89.78
Macau	84.38
San Marino	82.95
Andorra	82.36
Japan	82.17
Singapore	82.06
Hong Kong	81.96
Australia	81.72
Canada	81.29
France	81.09

Bottom 10 Countries	2010 Life Expectancy Estimate
South Africa	49.20
Guinea-Bissau	48.30
Chad	47.99
Swaziland	47.97
Zimbabwe	47.55
Nigeria	47.24
Afghanistan	44.65
Mozambique	41.37
Zambia	38.86
Angola	38.48

SOURCE: CIA World FactBook, "Life Expectancy at Birth," Estimate July 2010, www.cia.gov/library/publications/the-world-factbook/rankorder/2102rank.html?country Code=&rankAnchorRow=#.

extension may very well be viewed as something worth physically fighting over. The question, then, is twofold: will there be extended periods of time during which only wealthy members of society have access to longevity technologies, and if so, what options exist to ensure peace?

If we assume that technology divides will last a long time, as Canadian philosophy professor Christine Overall does, then it is worth considering as many potential outcomes as possible in order to prepare for what will certainly be a huge challenge. She predicts that enhancement technologies are likely to be "very scarce or extremely expensive."[41] Such a scenario, in which technology is attainable only by the rich and the poor have no hope of ever getting it, would create significant conflict. One way democratic societies might diffuse this tension, Fukuyama argues, is to allow the state to subsidize access to longevity technologies for the poor. Indeed, Overall suggests this same thing and argues that social justice requires giving longevity technology first to those "targeted by racial discrimination" as well as those who have suffered other injustices.[42] James Hughes, executive director of the Institute for Ethics and Emerging Technologies, makes a related argument, writing that any technology that "promises dramatic longevity or health" such that it "threatens social justice is an obvious candidate for subsidies and universal provision."[43] Although such suggestions for redistributing wealth might appeal to some, we have already seen how state subsidies for genetic enhancements could lead to worrisome eugenics programs. Instead of government control, an alternative is to free up markets and communication channels to the largest extent so that technology distribution can happen faster on its own. History shows that this is possible.

INNOVATION, EXPONENTIAL GROWTH, AND DISTRIBUTION OF TECHNOLOGY

New technologies are almost always adopted by the rich first, but over time they eventually reach everyone, and the historical record shows that the distribution of new technology is speeding up, not slowing down. In the book *Myths of Rich and Poor*, economist Michael Cox and author Richard Alm note that it took forty-six years for one-quarter of the population to get electricity and thirty-five years for the telephone to get that far. It took only sixteen years, however, for one-quarter of American households to get a personal computer, thirteen years for a cell phone, and seven years for Internet access, a promising trend for those who wish to see the widespread use of longevity technologies because health technologies are fast becoming information technologies.[44] As we learned in Chapter 2, genomics, which will help usher in personalized medicine, already shows positive signs because costs are dropping at lightning speeds.

"Biotech has gone exponential, like Moore's law," notes Andrew Hessel, a well-known synthetic biologist and cofounder of the Pink Army Cooperative, the world's first cooperative biotechnology company.[45] At the time of the writing of this book, advances in biotech were moving *faster* than Moore's law, according to which the number of transistors on an integrated circuit doubles approximately every two years. While the first Human Genome Project cost roughly *$2.7 billion* and Craig Venter spent about *$70 million* to sequence his own genome, by 2009 it was possible to get a genome sequenced for $5,000 and the $1,000 genome (or less) is in sight. Indeed, a partial DNA scan can already be had for only $199 at consumer genomics companies like 23andMe, and that company is using its data sets to attempt to link certain diseases to specific genes, important work on the way toward individually tailored pharmaceuticals and cures.[46]

Given the speed at which prices for new technology are shooting downward, particularly in biotechnology, the time horizon between longevity technology adoption by the rich and then by the poor *within* developed countries will probably shrink enough that few will consider taking up arms or unduly involving the state in repairing their bodies. As inventor Ray Kurzweil points out with extensive graphs and research, "The time gap between [those on the] leading and lagging edge is itself contracting."[47] And the time gap is not just dropping for obvious technological advancements like consumer electronics; it is also dropping in health technology. "AIDS drugs were about $30,000 per patient per year 15 years ago, and they didn't work very well," Kurzweil points out. "Now they actually work pretty well, and they're $100 per patient per year."[48]

Why is technology growing at an exponential rate? Kurzweil explains it through a theorem he calls the "Law of Accelerating Returns." Technology can move faster and faster, he explains, because "it builds on the fruits of the last stage."[49] Not only that, but there is also a positive feedback loop because "the more effective a particular evolutionary process becomes—for example, the higher the capacity and cost-effectiveness that computation attains—the greater the amount of resources that are deployed toward the further progress of that process."[50] Put simply, when humans see success, they tend to want to support it even more. It is also worth noting that such evolutionary systems are not closed and are usually improved by the chaos and diversity of the larger system. On this diversity point, Kurzweil's theory is supported by University of Michigan economist Scott E. Page, whose book *The Difference* explains that diverse groups of smart people are more likely than not to beat a single superintelligent person at problem solving because the group has the advantage of more than one perspective and group members can build on each other's ideas.[51]

Although advances in technology will move more quickly and be distributed to the masses faster than ever before, the rich will still have access to longevity medicines first. Cox and Alm explain why that's not necessarily a bad thing. They note that "virtually every new product requires an up-front investment, often sizeable, to cover the cost of getting started." The wealthy, who have the means to try new and expensive things, are thus the ones who "pay most of the new industries' early fixed costs—including research, plant and equipment, and market development."[52] There are many examples, from Queen Elizabeth owning some of the first silk stockings, to the rich paying $20 in 1915 for a three-minute phone call from New York to San

Francisco. Indeed, when genomics firm 23andMe (founded in 2006) first offered its DNA tests, the price was $1,000 for less information than is now available today at the $199 price. Two hundred dollars may still be too expensive for many Americans looking to understand their DNA, but the prices are only going to get cheaper (for continually better information) in short order. Given these realities, arguments that biotech shouldn't advance because the wealthy get it first are badly misinformed, if not outright immoral. In reality, it is the upfront investment from the wealthy that enables the masses to participate in whatever new innovations come along. Entrepreneurs are rarely successful by serving only the rich; economic growth happens when markets expand to include large numbers.

And if we are still nervous that technology might not move fast enough, let us consider the work of economist Paul Romer and author Matt Ridley. Romer became famous in the 1990s for advancing a theory that helped to explain why econometric models were so often wrong about economic growth. The reason, he argued, is that they don't take into account *ideas*—for example, the formula for a new drug or a novel way to produce customized computers.[53] As we learned in Chapter 3, ideas come from people, so the more people there are, the faster innovation happens, which in turn influences the wealth of the world. Matt Ridley builds upon Romer's theory and makes it more colorful. In his book *The Rational Optimist*, Ridley explains that "now the world is networked, and ideas are having sex with each other more promiscuously than ever, the pace of innovation will redouble and economic evolution will raise the living standards of the twenty-first century to unimagined heights, helping even the poorest of the world to afford to meet their desires as well as their needs."[54]

So far the evidence supports this premise: the more interconnected the growing (and free) world population becomes, the more opportunities there are for advancing innovation and moving it to a larger number of people. It is true, as Ridley points out, that "even if you break down the world into bits, it is hard to find any region that was worse off in 2005 than it was in 1955. . . . . The average South Korean lives twenty-six more years and earns fifteen times as much income each year as he did in 1955. The average Mexican lives longer now than the average Briton did in 1955."[55] These are not insignificant facts—they are the hallmarks of human progress driven by innovation and growth. And innovation can move forward only so long as people are free to share ideas and for-profit companies are able to make returns on their investments. As Romer argues, "The reality is that there are virtually no ideas which generate benefits for consumers if there's not an intervening for-profit firm which commercializes them, tailors them to the market, and then delivers them."[56] This means that we should celebrate when the wealthy want to spend their money helping new ideas get off the ground, and every effort should be made to create an environment where entrepreneurs can flourish. The market system is needed for new technologies to be both created and disbursed, and it would be tragic as well as morally wrong to stand in the way of this growth for any of the reasons covered in this chapter.

WOULD OUR ANCESTORS
HAVE WANTED TO LIVE LONGER?

No one argues that humans *already* live too long. If we went back in time to 1850, when life expectancy was around forty-three years, and asked people if it would be good to live longer, the optimists would have said yes and the pessimists would have declared the possibility a disaster. Who would want to live longer, they would have said, when life was so hard? There was no electricity, so families would have warmed themselves at the fire, inhaling smoke that caused a chronic cough. Most people worked at a grueling physical job, and living longer would have meant only seeing more friends die of infectious diseases or in childbirth. Life was boring, since few people would have had much education or access to leisure and entertainment. And many would have worried that injecting themselves with strange things called vaccines to fight disease would have made them less human. "God wouldn't want that, and we shouldn't either" might have been the consensus.

Today, such an argument seems ridiculous because advances in knowledge of all kinds have made the world a better place. No one is less human because of scientific and technological discoveries, not even those people who have "fake ears" (hearing aids) or "fake limbs" (prosthetics). Life expectancy is projected to keep climbing, but how the multitude of upcoming new technologies will make our lives better and more rewarding is not yet known. Few could have predicted the Internet's arrival, yet in just over a decade it has changed and enriched our lives in many ways. As philosopher Max More puts it, "If there were, in principle, some limit to the length of a stimulating, challenging, rewarding life, we could not know where it lies until we reached it."[57] We haven't reached it yet, and it is unlikely that we will anytime soon.

Now that we have tackled many of the objections to living longer, it is time to consider how life will change once health spans actually expand. One of the most important areas of potential change, the family, is the topic of the next chapter.

CHAPTER 5

The Changing Face of Family

O N NOVEMBER 28, 2008, a woman named Rajo Devi gave birth to a baby girl in India. Like many couples who have had problems conceiving, Devi and her husband were thrilled that their use of reproductive technology led to the birth of a healthy baby. "We longed for a child all these years and now we are very happy to have one," she told reporters.[1] This reads like a common success story, as millions of couples turn to medical science for help with fertility issues, but in this case Devi was seventy years old when she gave birth. The response from commentators was swift.

"Ms. Devi's newborn can be called a triumph of science over infertility, but is this really a triumph?" wondered family author Lisa Belkin in the *New York Times*.[2] "If 70 isn't too old to become a mom or dad, what is?" asked *Slate*'s William Saletan.[3] These are good questions that require thoughtful answers because Devi and her husband (then seventy-two) are not the only older parents to produce a baby and they certainly won't be the last.

Of course, men have always been able to have children at late ages. Charlie Chaplin was seventy-three when his youngest son was born and, more recently, Rupert Murdoch was seventy-two when his third wife gave birth to daughter Chloe.[4] Now that science makes it possible for women to join men in procreating at older ages, more than a few eyebrows have been raised and not just in the media. For instance,

Italy's Association of Medical Practitioners and Dentists barred their members from administering fertility treatments to women over fifty, and a former health minister of France, Dr. Philippe Douste-Blazy, argued that "artificial late pregnancies were immoral as well as dangerous to the health of mother and child. . . . [He] urged women not to be 'egoistic' by trying to become pregnant after menopause."[5] Such statements might make some feminists fume, but if life expectancy is around 80 years, then having a baby at age 70 means that the parent is likely to die when the child is still very young. Indeed, such a scenario played out with Carmen Bousada, who gave birth to twin boys at age 66 and then died two years later of stomach cancer.[6] Bousada was unfortunately ahead of her time in thinking that she would live long enough to take care of her kids. Her own mother had lived to be 101 years, prompting Bousada to tell reporters after the births, "If I live as long as my mom did, imagine, I could even have grandchildren."[7] But such expectations may someday be realistic. As we have seen, exponentially growing technologies are set to radically increase life expectancy.

As it stands now, most women are infertile by age fifty. Those who have given birth after this age have done so mainly by using a combination of reproductive technologies and donated eggs and sperm. Even though current fertility treatments can allow an older mother to act as a surrogate—that is, carry a younger, donated egg to term—a woman's own eggs still tend to expire sometime around age forty to fifty.[8] To be clear, both Rajo Devi and Carmen Bousada gave birth at old ages, but the children they produced were not biologically theirs. This fact would make pregnancy at an older age undesirable for many women and leads us to the obvious first question concerning family in a book on health span extension: can biological fertility be extended along with life expectancy?

FERTILITY TECHNOLOGY TODAY AND BEYOND

In 1978 Dr. Howard Jones and Dr. Georgeanna Jones, two reproductive specialists who were also husband and wife, thought they were going to retire. Georgeanna had been director of the Laboratory of Reproductive Physiology at Johns Hopkins University, and Howard had been the director of the university's International Program on Fertility Control.[9] Because the university had a mandatory retirement age of sixty-five, the aging doctors packed up and moved to Norfolk, Virginia, to teach at the new Eastern Virginia Medical School and to start making plans for retirement. Then something big changed their direction.

On July 25, 1978, Louise Brown, the world's first "test-tube" baby, was born in England through the help of in vitro fertilization (IVF). IVF is a method whereby eggs are removed from the ovaries, fertilized outside the woman's body, and then placed in the woman's uterus, bypassing the need for fallopian tubes. According to reports, a local journalist asked Howard Jones if a test tube baby would be possible in the United States.

"Yes," he answered, but "it would take some money." Not long after, he received a call from a former patient offering the funds to open an IVF clinic, which he and Georgeanna accepted. With the help of both Howard and Georgeanna Jones, on December 28, 1981, America's first test tube baby, Elizabeth Jordan Carr, was born.[10] The procedure to create this pregnancy was the first in the world to use a stimulated gonadotropin cycle, that is, the ability to induce the development of multiple eggs.[11] This advancement by the Joneses was a major breakthrough that has allowed thousands of otherwise infertile couples to produce healthy children. It is notable that one of America's great advances in reproductive technology was created by two doctors late in their own lives. The pair helped to bring thousands of babies into the world and were considered "third grandparents" by many of the children aided by their clinic.[12]

What started as a pioneering idea has now turned into a very big business. Over the last two decades or so, fertility clinics have mushroomed across America and the world. By 1996 there were 302 clinics in the United States, and by 2006 there were 483.[13] Scores of new patients have kept the "baby business" booming—the number of assisted reproductive technology cycles begun each year has more than doubled since 1996 (64,681 cycles in 1996 versus 138,198 in 2006), and the total tally of successful live birth deliveries has nearly tripled in that time.[14]

Although improving the chances for women over forty to become pregnant and give birth, IVF does not guarantee that outcome; as medical researchers noted in a major report released January 2009, "IVF does not reverse the clock."[15] Annual data from fertility clinics show that the percentage of IVF procedures resulting in live births using embryos from a woman's own eggs declines dramatically with the advancing age of the mother.[16] However, because egg donors are typically in their twenties or early thirties, the health of many of the eggs are intact, and as a result the percentage of live births resulting from donor eggs remains consistently high for women throughout their forties.[17] Yet many older women are unwilling to use donor eggs, and this will likely still be the case when humans expand their life expectancy even further. Clinics are aware of this fact, and already techniques have been created that give women the option to have their own eggs frozen and stored for use at a later date.

Although "egg freezing" is offered by many fertility clinics now, the survival rates are low, and cryopreservation of healthy eggs and tissue for reproductive procedures is still considered experimental. Sperm and embryos have been successfully frozen for decades, but freezing unfertilized eggs is still a delicate and difficult process. Eggs are filled with a high water content, so once frozen, large ice crystals can form that destroy the eggs' cellular structure.

Much of the scientific activity on extending fertility is aimed at aiding women who have survived breast cancer, ovarian cancer, and other diseases that require chemotherapy and radiotherapy that rendered them sterile. Fertility clinics have now begun experimenting with new "vitrification" techniques to improve the preservation rates of healthy eggs. For instance, researchers at the Colorado Center for Reproductive Medicine (CCRM) have refined a process of egg freezing using liquid nitrogen that, according to CCRM, has produced "egg survival rates of approximately 80%, fertilization rates over 80%, and pregnancy rates above 50%."[18]

New techniques to extend the reproductive functioning of ovaries have also been explored in recent years. For example, in November 2008 the first birth from a full ovary transplant was announced to the public, a promising sign for older women who are unable to conceive owing to menopause, cancer treatment, or other causes of ovarian failure.[19] In this case, a thirty-eight-year-old woman from London who experienced ovarian failure in her teenage years, sending her into early menopause, received an ovary from her twin sister. This procedure could pave the way for more women to have ovaries removed and frozen along with their eggs, to be thawed later on when they choose to have a child. Another procedure transplants only parts of ovarian tissue.

In February 2007, a Danish woman, Stinne Holm Bergholdt, gave birth to a baby girl after receiving a transplant of six strips of her own ovarian tissue that she had had frozen in 2004 before she underwent chemotherapy for bone cancer. The cancer treatment put her into early menopause, but in 2005 doctors transplanted her tissue back into her body and her ovaries started to work again. Her 2007 pregnancy was helped along by IVF, but to her surprise in January 2008 she learned that she had become pregnant again naturally.[20] After delivering her second baby, in September 2008, she became the first woman to have two children following an ovarian tissue transplant.[21] As of this writing, around the world there have already been close to ten instances of children being born owing to ovarian tissue transplants. The techniques described so far rely on early preplanning, so for those who want to start a family later in life, there is a need for raising awareness of the options.

But do women really want to have children as they get older, particularly because the onset of advanced age has traditionally brought a higher probability of pregnancy complications, miscarriages, and child disabilities? For many women, the answer is yes because despite these risks more women are already waiting longer before becoming first-time mothers. According to the Centers for Disease Control and Prevention (CDC), the average age of first-time mothers in America has steadily increased over the last four decades, from 21.4 years in 1970 to 25 years in 2006.[22] More importantly, the proportion of first births to women aged thirty-five years and older increased by nearly eightfold from 1970 to 2006. That's a big change, showing the growing desire of women to have children later than was historically the case.

The era of the forty-year-old new mom is already beginning, even before significant life-extension technologies hit the market. Data from the CDC's National Vital Statistics Reports indicate that the number of births to U.S. women in their forties more than doubled from 1990 to 2006, from 50,245 to 112,019 births.[23] Surprisingly, this jump occurred while the growth in nationwide births rose only marginally overall, from 4,158,212 births in 1990 to 4,265,555 births in 2006. And it's not just American women who are pushing this trend forward. In general, there has been a doubling in the number of live births to women over forty across the countries of the Organisation for Economic Co-operation and Development (OECD) over a span of about fifteen years (see Figure 5.1).[24]

As life expectancy increases, the age at which women will want to have children will likely continue to grow, thereby increasing demand for reproductive technology to add even more time to women's biological clocks. Aside from egg freezing and ovarian transplants, what other technologies might help older parents-to-be conceive in the future? Are there any technologies that might remove the need to preplan or at least make preplanning an easier and cheaper process?

One possibility that could really change the rules of the game is the ability to grow eggs in the lab. This would entail taking tiny pieces of ovarian tissue through keyhole surgery, a minimally invasive technique that is less painful and requires less recovery time than regular surgery. The tissue, which contains thousands of immature eggs, would be frozen until the woman decided to have children, at which point scientists would stimulate the eggs in the lab to grow to the point where

FIGURE 5.1

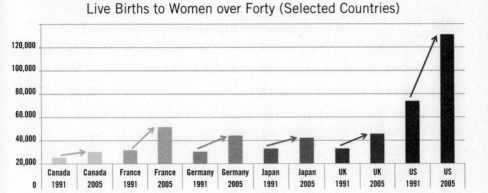

Live Births to Women over Forty (Selected Countries)

they could be fertilized. This method would allow women to avoid injecting themselves with hormones or having to undergo an uncomfortable procedure to harvest mature eggs. If science makes it easier and less painful for women to extend their biological clocks, it won't just be outliers like Rajo Devi or Carmen Bousada who have children much later in life. Many women may ultimately choose this path, marking the beginning of the era of the 70-year-old mom. Today, that sounds strange, but in a world with 150-year life expectancies, it could be commonplace.

If growing eggs in the lab seems far off, consider that it has already been successfully completed with both mouse and human tissue. In the case of the mouse, it led to a successful pregnancy and live birth.[25] When it comes to the human experiment, researchers have demonstrated that they can mature the eggs in the lab and they were (at the time of this writing) simply waiting for an appropriate candidate who desired to take it to a full pregnancy at a fertility clinic.[26] According to fertility researcher Dr. Teresa Woodruff of Northwestern University, the breakthrough that finally allowed scientists to mature the human eggs was a "hydrogel called alginate, which doesn't touch or contact the (ovarian) follicle cells but just supports them."[27] With many women currently looking to preserve their fertility before undergoing cancer treatment, it shouldn't be long before a human case is put to the test.

Although men's biological clocks do not tick as loudly, they do tick, and research shows that the older a man is, the more likely it is that his sperm will lead to problems like autism and bipolar disorder, as well as plain ineffectiveness.[28] Fertility researchers are therefore also investigating new techniques to enhance male fertility.

In July 2009 British researchers announced that they were able to create human sperm cells from stem cells.[29] Although such a development is not shocking given the transformative nature of stem cells, there is still much work to be done as the cells that were created were not identical to natural sperm cells and therefore would not likely have created an embryo. Even so, the fact that scientists have been able to create spermlike cells means that growing functional sperm for men who are infertile may become possible. Clearly, a path is being paved that will allow both women and men to have biological children at even later ages if they wish. This means that both biological and nonbiological fertility will be extended at the same time as health spans increase. The next question, then, is, how will this ability affect marriage and family creation?

GETTING AROUND TO "I DO"

It's no secret that there is already a trend among young people toward later marriage. According to the U.S. Census Bureau, the age at first marriage has been on the rise for decades, and today the median age is twenty-eight years for men and twenty-six years for women, an increase of 22 percent and 30 percent for men and women, respectively, since 1950.[30] The reasons for this increase are often attributed to a combination of factors, including a "career-first, marriage-later" approach that has become more common for young people, particularly women. Indeed, the U.S. Department of Labor reports that women now make up 46 percent of the total U.S. labor force, with almost 40 percent of all working women holding jobs in management, professional, or specialty occupations that require advanced degrees and years of training.[31] In addition, most women these days are active in the labor force (60 percent), whereas only 30 percent of women were actively employed outside the home forty years ago.[32]

The phenomenon of women seeking independence before marriage is becoming so commonplace that University of Texas, Austin sociologist Mark Regnerus worries that "many women report feeling peer pressure to avoid giving serious thought to marriage until they're at least in their late 20s."[33] If a woman is seeking a mate in college, Regnerus argues, she is "considered a pariah, someone after her 'Mrs. degree.'"[34] Of course, it's not only women who are looking to establish themselves before getting married.

Research published by the MacArthur Foundation Network on Transitions to Adulthood at the University of Pennsylvania sums up the cultural transition on marriage nicely: "where once being married meant you were an adult, today you have to be an adult to be married."[35] Essentially, marriage is no longer expected to cause the disappearance of the individual. Instead, it is now viewed as "something akin to a pair of choreographed figure skaters. Each partner moves on the ice separately, and yet each one must always be aware of the other, somehow managing to move in tandem."[36]

The individuals who ascribe to this now-popular view of marriage are labeled "marriage planners" by Saint Joseph University sociology professor Maria Kefalas and her colleagues. The planners, they argue, "are inclined to regard marriage as a developmental process which progresses over time and is tested by real-life circumstances."[37] This is in contrast to a small minority Dr. Kefalas calls "marriage drifters," who "continue to think of marriage as inevitable and a natural outcome of an early and untested relationship."[38] That Dr. Kefalas and her colleagues make a distinction based on planning brings the concept of time into clear focus. That is, with greater longevity, individuals have more time. The average life expectancy in 1850 was around forty-three years, so individuals did not have the luxury of waiting around to look for their "perfect soul mate." The goal instead was to have children early and hope for the best.

Now that life expectancy is around eighty years, young people can focus on economic stability and other important life elements before committing to someone "until death do us part." In other words, men and women are already delaying marriage in large part because they know they have more time in their lives in which to have a family, so they are taking that time to properly plan and select a mate. The increase in life expectancy also helps to explain the growing number of people who cohabit, or live together, without being married.

Cohabitation took off as a trend following the sexual revolution in the 1960s that made sex outside marriage acceptable. According to David Popenoe, codirector of the National Marriage Project at Rutgers University, "As of 2002, over 50 percent of women ages 19 to 44 had cohabited for a portion of their lives, compared to 33 percent in 1987 and virtually none a hundred years ago."[39] However, if cohabitation hadn't kick-started with the sexual revolution, it would have happened anyway in response to longer life expectancies. That's because it is a relationship structure that allows individuals to be in a serious relationship without being forced to make a premature lifelong commitment. Waiting until the time is right works in tandem with planning a marriage that is more likely to be stable and happy; couples have time to figure out who they are and what kind of relationship is best for them. It makes sense, then, that sociologists report the surprising-to-some finding that, although more people are marrying later and cohabiting, most people still believe in and aspire to join the institution of marriage.[40]

MORE TIME ON THE ROAD TO ADULTHOOD

Delayed marriage and cohabitation are the most-discussed results of our already expanded life expectancy, but there are also some less-obvious outcomes that are beginning to emerge and have only recently been explored by scholars and the popular media. For instance, human life is often viewed in phases, such as childhood, adolescence, adulthood, and old age. Lengthening of life expectancies, along with changing economic circumstances and gender equality, has begun to usher in a new phase of life between adolescence and adulthood. In 2002 *Newsweek* called individuals in this phase of life "adultolescents." Linda Perlman Gordon and Susan Morris Shaffer, authors of *Mom, Can I Move Back in with You?* call the phase "adultescence."[41]

Whatever the name for this phase, it's apparent that young people today no longer make a clear transition from adolescence to adulthood around the "traditional" ages of eighteen to twenty. Dr. Jeffrey Jensen Arnett, psychology professor at the University of Maryland and author of *Emerging Adulthood*, explains the situation this way: "it takes longer to get to adulthood than it did 40 years ago, but maybe that's a good thing. Maybe they'll have a better shot at happiness than all the people who got married at 20 and divorced."[42] He's probably right because research on divorce shows clearly that those who get married at older ages tend to stay married. As Rutgers University anthropologist Dr. Helen Fisher puts it, "Divorce is for the young." In her book *Anatomy of Love*, she notes that "eighty-one percent of all divorces occur before age 45 among women; 74 percent of all divorces happen before age 45 among men."[43] Most divorce, she reports, happens when people are in their twenties.[44] And it's not just age that affects the divorce rate. Education is also a factor. Research conducted by Betsey Stevenson of the Wharton School at the University of Pennsylvania shows that "the lowest divorce rates are among people who marry late with more education; the highest ones are among those who marry young with less education."[45] Of course, as humans live longer, they will have more opportunities for higher education, so divorce rates could be expected to decline.

So what exactly are young people doing during their adultescence? It's not that young people are "unwilling to take on adult roles," argue noted sociologists Frank F. Furstenberg, Rubén G. Rumbaut, and Richard A. Settersten. Instead, the reality is that "pathways into adulthood have grown more varied and complex. Once, youth moved nearly in lockstep through the stages that mark adulthood. Now, they alternate or simultaneously pursue education and work, cycle between periods living at home and living independently, and delay marriage and parenting."[46]

An excellent firsthand account of this new complexity is given in Ethan Watters's book *Urban Tribes*, in which he explains that during this period of transition a person's friends substitute for family in urban centers across the country as young people get educated, begin to develop their careers by working long hours, and learn more about their interests. Two key ideas are worth considering from Watters's book. First, the freedom that comes with having more time in early adulthood has allowed his generation to learn more about themselves before committing to starting a family.[47] Second, he and his peers have become more comfortable with their respective identities as a result.[48]

Clearly, longer life expectancies have already changed the transition to adulthood, which raises the question of whether extending life expectancy further will extend the adultescence phase or create a new one. Predicting the future isn't easy, but we can safely say that adultescence will remain and become more widely recognized. There may even be new phases of life in the later years because, as we learned in Chapter 2, life extension in the future will come from adding years to the end of life, not the beginning, as was the case previously. Sociologist Dr. William Sadler argues that a new phase of life he calls the "third age" has already begun and is due to a "30-year life bonus" that previous generations didn't have.[49] His organization, the Center for Third Age Leadership, tells visitors to its Web site that in the third age "advancement becomes less important" and "wisdom and self-awareness bring new ease with ourselves and others."[50] Whether or not this phase will remain common as more people delay childbearing into later ages remains to be seen, but there will always be some who decide to have children earlier than others, and in those cases a phase like the third age may exist. We can say for sure that the most significant result of having a longer life, and therefore more time, is having more options—to have children early or late, get married early or late, and so on. Such choice will create more diversity when it comes to individual growth and types of relationships.

THE EVOLUTION OF FAMILY: COUPLE RELATIONSHIPS AND CHILDREN

With an average life expectancy of 150 years, great age differences, say eighty or ninety years, between partners might occur. Nevertheless, the historical evidence suggests that such relationships probably won't be common, regardless of the good health of the older partner. The last time humans significantly extended their life expectancy, the average age difference between partners didn't change much.

Detailed research from Statistics Norway indicates that the total number of couples with large age differences between the partners did not significantly increase between 1906 and 2002.[51] The basic age difference remained at around 3.5 years (men being slightly older), and this was common across the OECD. There were, however, some changes over time. For instance, in 1996, 6 percent of men were more than ten years older than their partners, and this increased to 12 percent in 2002. Across the same period, the percentage of women ten years older than their partners changed from 1 to 3 percent.[52] In the United States, data for New Jersey in 2003 indicate that 10.1 percent of marriages involved a man ten years older than his spouse and only 2.3 percent of marriages involved a woman at least ten years older than her spouse.[53]

Social responses to large age differences between partners are often either censorious or prurient, which is perhaps one reason that these types of relationships are limited. For instance, much media attention was given to a survey that indicated that men were more likely to be unfaithful if their partner was more than ten years older.[54] In this case, the commentary was framed as a warning to women to avoid this type of relationship and to take extra care to maintain the relationships they had. Similar comments are less frequently made about men in the same situation.[55]

Will the number of men marrying much younger women continue to grow as such relationships become less stigmatized? If, as researchers at Stanford, the University of California, Santa Barbara, and the University of Wisconsin argue, older men seek younger partners primarily to continue having children, such men won't need to find younger partners once it is easier for older women to have their own biological children using fertility technologies.[56] Large-age-difference relationships will probably also remain uncommon because we tend to seek partners with whom we have significant things in common—education level, professional roles, and age.[57] And in the future older women (and men) will likely look less "aged" because they will remain healthy for much longer periods of time, so remarriage for beauty or "youth" will lose some of its distinguishing force. As noted above, even though the data show an increase in the percentage of relationships with an age difference of ten or more years as life expectancy has grown, the raw numbers still remain small.

Although getting married later may work to reduce the frequency of divorce as people choose more suitable partners, more time to live also raises the possibility of more breakups and remarriages. Today, some people get married two or even three times, but as people live longer, those numbers could increase, and for at least a small slice of the population they could hit (or exceed) Elizabeth Taylor proportions.[58] An interesting consequence of greater longevity is a higher incidence of serial monogamy regardless of whether it leads to marriage, perhaps interspersed with periods of living alone. The "urban tribes" Ethan Watters describes may commonly exist not only during adultescence but also during other stages of life in which an individual is single. Thus, a key question emerges: will longevity lead to longer relationships or more relationships? A pragmatic answer is both. Human beings seem able to seek and sustain an almost infinite range of relationships to provide companionship, comfort, a means to bring up children, and sexual pleasure. As Cornell University anthropologist Meredith Small nicely puts it, "We don't always form nuclear families in the ideal way, but we do make families of a different order all the time, because it's human nature to be together."[59]

Against this background, the most likely outcome of increased health spans is a far higher diversity of practical living arrangements and of relationships between the individuals currently grouped into family units. And once we add children to the mix, the potential for longevity to generate a wide range of family structures increases even more.

One obvious result of extended fertility and life expectancy will be growth in the ranks of older parents. Most of the research on older parents points out that the main disadvantages are that they tend to be less energetic than younger parents (and, of course, closer to death). However, in a world where people remain healthy for much longer periods of time, this downside will disappear and the upsides of being an older parent, such as greater financial stability, higher levels of confidence, and more patience, will remain and benefit children.[60] Another criticism of older parents, according to Ohio State associate professor of family and consumer sciences Nancy Recker, is that "older parents can put a lot of pressure on their children to succeed, to be a super achiever."[61] The research on this point is not extensive, however, and it may simply be that today's older parents are selected for a certain personality type, which will not necessarily be the case in the future.

Perhaps a more interesting possible change resulting from the ability to have children at later ages is very large age gaps between siblings. At the moment, it is relatively rare to have an age gap of more than twenty years between children of the same biological parents. If the gap is greater than that, the new child is usually a consequence of the biological father remarrying and starting what is effectively a second family. In a future of extended health spans and reproductive time, the possibility for large age differences among siblings mushrooms. For instance, siblings could be separated by two years, twenty years, or even fifty or seventy years. This raises the question of how age gaps between children change their intrafamily

relationships and how this might promote conflict or closeness between siblings.[62]

A popular view is that siblings born close together appear to fight
more in childhood but tend to be closer as adults. Even though it
is true that siblings of the same age group have a more meaningful
and longer-lasting relationship than those separated by more years,
whether the siblings will have a positive relationship depends on
other factors, such as personality.[63] However, siblings of a similar age
clearly help to socialize each other because they spend more time
playing together. According to researchers at Concordia University in
Canada, "As youngsters spend large amounts of time playing together,
they know each other very well. This long history and intimate
knowledge translates into opportunities for providing emotional and
instrumental support for one another."[64] Indeed, some evidence suggests that children born relatively far apart tend to live very separate
lives with limited interaction.[65] But it is also true that elder siblings
can help younger children cope with stress and manage their external
relationships.[66] It all depends on how far apart the siblings are, what
their personalities are like, and how close the family members are in
general. Of course, siblings fifty to seventy years apart don't yet exist,
so it is difficult to predict how the relationship would function, but it
probably would be closer to that of a child-aunt/uncle or even child-
grandparent. With potentially large age differences between parents
and children and siblings, the question of family culture also arises.

FAMILY CULTURE AND SHARED MEMORIES

A common finding among research psychologists is that groups
(families, coworkers, leisure clubs, etc.) tend to develop a shared
identity from stories and memories.[67] We tend to choose friends and
partners on the basis of similarity, and we tend to feel more identifi-
cation with a group with which we share some of the stories and
narratives that give the group its definition.[68] These stories are then
used to interpret future events, and their repetition and elaboration

are a crucial element in group formation and maintenance.[69] In a
family setting, such stories have a structure like this:

"Do you remember when? . . ."

"You used to? . . ."

What happens, then, to shared stories in families where there are
greater age gaps? Will grandparents and great-grandparents help
keep family ties strong, or will age gaps contribute to a weakened
sense of family culture?

The sibling research just discussed revealed that increased age
differences could lead to more distant relationships. One reason for
this might be fewer opportunities for shared narratives, and even
when an event was shared, the participants could see it very differ-
ently. A fictional representation of this phenomenon is provided in
Ian Rankin's novel A *Question of Blood*:

"Remember that day you took me to the park?"

"The day we played football?"

"You remember it? . . . We were playing football and some guys
you knew turned up. . . . Then we started walking home. Or you and
your pals did, me trailing behind, carrying the ball. . . . We were
passing [a pub] only then you turned, pointed at me, told me I'd
have to wait outside. Your voice was different, a lot harder, like you
didn't want your pals to know we were pals. . . . You didn't come out
and I knew I couldn't go in. . . . You never asked what had happened
to the ball, and I knew why you didn't ask . . . because it wasn't important to you. . . . And I was just some little kid again and not your
friend."

Rebus was trying to remember. . . . The day he'd thought he'd
known had been sunshine and football.[70]

The dialogue between these two men, one in his late fifties and
his cousin in his forties, shows how age can affect perception of certain events. Indeed, not only age but also the generation into which
a person is born can influence perspective. Consider moments that

are iconic to certain generations. The shooting of President John F. Kennedy in 1963 or the terrorist attacks of September 11, 2001, are examples of events that most people recall (even if they differ in their interpretation of meaning and understanding). Such shared events and memories are part of the social fabric that holds together groups of people as families, communities, and even nations.[71]

One effect of greater longevity will be a reduction in the proportion of people who have shared particular events and, even if shared, see them from roughly the same viewpoint. Thus, siblings who differed by forty or more years or individuals who had 110-year-old parents would have quite different perspectives from their family members and could potentially have a more difficult time bridging the gaps. That said, not all parents would choose to create such large age differences within their families (perhaps for this reason), and the shared culture of some families might be so strong that the age gaps wouldn't matter quite as much.

For example, Columbia psychology professor E. Tory Higgins has identified how our views of someone else (and the extent to which we see that person as being important) strongly influence our overall interaction. More importantly, after a group achieves a shared language and shared memories, Dr. Higgins argues, "the shared reality created by the group survives across generations of subjects, indicating that once a shared reality is achieved, it can be maintained with stability long after the originators of the norm have gone."[72] What does this mean for the communication of a family's values and beliefs?

Ute Schönpflug, a German expert in developmental psychology at Martin Luther University, argues that there is no simplistic process for transmitting social and attitudinal values, but that parenting style and education have an impact. She writes, "The transmission of values requires competence on the part of the parents to use transmission strategies (e.g., communication in a family discussion) to convince their offspring to internalize certain values."[73] This suggests that as individuals become more educated, a likelihood in a longer-lived society, communication between generations may become easier than it would be otherwise. Nevertheless, some children, and not just during adolescence, fundamentally reject their parents' values.

How vast age divides will affect the ability to transfer family values and culture will depend on the size of the gaps and the level of communication between members of the family. Those families with the largest age gaps may see a reduction in their role as a means to create and transmit certain values and memories across generations. As with so much else in the debate over longevity and the family, this is not necessarily good or bad—but it will be different. Families with extreme generation divides may have to be extra resourceful in their quest to create and sustain shared memories and values.

FAMILY SIZE AND STRUCTURE

Since the 1950s, the industrialized world has seen a steady decline in the number of children per adult of childbearing age. Demographers generally argue that this is a product of increasing wealth, access to contraception (especially after the wider availability of the contraceptive pill in the early 1960s), greater female participation in the workforce, and improved child mortality rates. Table 5.1 documents the clear drop in the number of children per adult female across a number of OECD member states as gross domestic product (GDP) has grown.[74]

One of the concerns often cited about falling birthrates is the danger that the population will shrink once it falls beneath the rate needed to sustain itself, about 2.1 children per adult female. On this basis, all the countries listed in the table will see population decline, although that decrease will happen more slowly once people begin to live longer (because death rates will shrink). Indeed, if birthrates do not go up, the discussion about age gaps between siblings will be slightly less important because there will be more only children born to each pair of biological parents. The population could shrink even further if the number of people choosing not to have children at all increases.

TABLE 5.1

GDP Per Capita and Changing Family Size

Country	GDP Per Capita 1950	Number of Children 1950	GDP Per Capita 2000	Number of Children 2000
Australia	7,412	3.18	21,605	1.76
Canada	7,291	3.65	22,360	1.52
Italy	3,502	2.32	18,774	1.29
Netherlands	5,996	3.06	22,161	1.73
Sweden	6,739	2.21	20,710	1.67
United Kingdom	6,939	2.18	20,353	1.70
United States	9,561	3.45	28,449	2.04

Some futurists have implied that as people live longer, the rate of childlessness may increase. For instance, aging theorist Aubrey de Grey argues that "our presumption that there is this innate drive to have kids, quite often, may not be so strong as we may have been brought up to believe."[75] The idea is that women (and men) may be so satisfied with their lives (careers, relationships, travel) that they will keep putting off having children until they finally decide that they don't really need to have children in order to live fulfilling lives. This might sound like a strange theory to some, but there is already a movement of activists promoting "childfree" lives. One Web site devoted to the cause explains that "we choose to call ourselves 'childfree' rather than 'childless,' because we feel the term 'childless' implies that we're missing something we want—and we aren't. We consider ourselves childFREE—free of the loss of personal freedom, money, time and energy that having children requires."[76]

A typical reaction to such strong antichild sentiments is that they must be the result of some childhood trauma or personality quirk, but extensive research on the subject shows that those who choose a childfree life are simply "less apt to view children as bringing rewards in important life areas."[77] Raising children does take a lot of time, hard work, and financial resources. Because children are no longer seen as an economic benefit, which they were when labor was needed on the family farm, the main benefit these days is in the form of community. So perhaps the best way to think about whether the childfree movement will gain ground as humans extend their lives is to consider whether the love, friendship, and joy of children can be replaced by longer-term relationships with adults.

It is unlikely that adults will substitute for the role of children for most people. Children are special because they actually share biological traits with their parents, they are molded by their parents from the beginning, and this can't be replicated any other way. Indeed, although the ranks of the childless are larger than they were thirty years ago (possibly owing to women waiting too long to have children), the percentage of the population that *chooses* this lifestyle seems to have leveled off.[78] According to the CDC/National Center for Health Statistics, in 1995 the percentage of women *voluntarily* choosing to be childless was 6.6 percent; in 2002 (the last available year for this data) the percentage of women who made this choice was 6.2 percent.[79]

Humans are social beings after all, and as science and technology allow us to live longer and healthier lives, family may actually become *more* important because such relationships will fill more years than ever before. Also, as our lives become longer, the amount of time we spend on the hard work of raising children will become a smaller percentage of our lives, perhaps making the burden seem less intense. How would such a theory fit with the data showing a preference for fewer children as societies become more wealthy and longer-lived?

As society continues to get richer, fertility is generally expected to continue declining even further, but research conducted at the University of Pennsylvania shows that is not a guaranteed outcome. According to Dr. Mikko Myrskylä and his colleagues, once the development of a country reaches a certain level, the fertility rate starts to rise again (see Figure 5.2).[80]

FIGURE 5.2

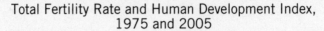

Total Fertility Rate and Human Development Index,
1975 and 2005

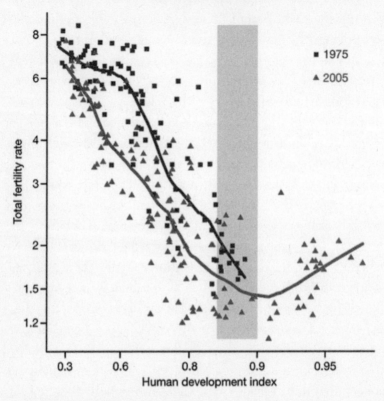

SOURCE: Mikko Myrskylä, Hans-Peter Kohler, and Francesco C. Billari, "Advances in Development Reverse Fertility Declines," *Nature* 460, 741–743, August 6, 2009. Copyright 2009 *Nature Magazine*. Reprinted by permission of Macmillan Publishers, Ltd.

"Development" in this case takes into account wealth, education, and longevity. What accounts for the increase in the number of children once societies are more highly developed needs further investigation, but a good hypothesis does exist. Ecologists have noted that when environments are unstable, it is reproductively strategic to have many children with the hope that at least some of them will survive. When environments become stable, however, the strategy can shift to having a smaller number of children on whom parents dote, making sure that they have every possible advantage. Therefore, as societies make the transition from developing to developed, the number of children shrinks as parents can afford to spend a lot of resources on only one or two kids. As those societies continue to get wealthier, however, parents can afford to have even more children and still spend large amounts of resources on them.

So it seems that, although fertility rates initially trend down with growing wealth and longevity, they could go up again (at least a bit) as development continues to increase. But even if that doesn't happen, greater longevity and more time to access reproductive technologies will cause families to become more complex and varied.

A RETURN TO EXTENDED AND MIXED FAMILIES

Extended and mixed families are not new, and the concept of a single marital relationship for life is a relatively recent event. Previously, the main cause of marriage breakup was not intent (divorce) but early mortality (death in childbirth, disease, industrial accident, war, etc.), and remarriage with existing children or adoption of orphaned children was common.[81] Historically, then, it's been relatively common for children to be brought up socially with one or both of their biological parents absent.[82] The reasons for forming new family structures are often a mix of the economic and the social.

A study by sociology professors Cheryl Elman and Andrew London sheds light on remarriage at the turn of the twentieth century. They write that "remarriage generally provided a means to augment economic or instrumental domestic supports," but that there were differences between women and men in their reasons for tying the knot a second time.[83] Whereas "women were less likely than men to remarry and tended to use remarriage as a means to obtain income support," men "tended to remarry for immediate instrumental assistance with children and household management, allowing them to continue their economic activities."[84]

Adoption also occurred for economic reasons, but it was governed by local norms and laws. For instance, historian Witold Kula points to a Polish judicial writ from the year 1729 that says, "If it happens that a couple dies, whose husband is a farm-hand in the service of a peasant, it is the duty of the peasant to bring up their children. If a childless neighbor offers to take one of them at his home, he shall be allowed to."[85] Taking in orphans was a fast way to grow a family or replace children who had died early. Such a strategy was economically expedient; the more hands there were, the more work could be done.

Because adoption was common in remarriage as well as in situations in which children lost their parents, a common family arrangement included those with nonbiological ties and a greater number of members of different ages and relationships. In the future longer lives combined with new reproductive technologies and divorce could lead to more family relationships based on social links rather than biological kinship, returning families back to these older social structures.

Today, we have already witnessed how divorce and remarriage result in individuals belonging to more than one family group, often causing complications during the holidays when older children must decide which "set of parents" to visit on which day. Stepparents, stepsiblings, and even stepgrandparents have become relatively common. Australian data indicate that around 40 percent of Australian remarriages involve one or both members of the new couple already having children under sixteen.[86] Research into the relationships between children and adults in a family setting in which one or both adults have left their previous partners indicates that there can be considerable difficulties in dealing with the new social structure and in being members of more than one family. Marriage and family therapy professor Joan D. Atwood explains that "blending two families is an inherently disorganizing experience that involves a total transformation of the individuals' world. There is a lack of a common history and therefore a lack of a common culture."[87] Anyone who has been through this experience knows it can be very difficult, but the good news is that the evidence shows that these difficulties are not universal and sometimes relatively short-lived.[88]

With longer lives and new reproductive technologies, the number and diversity of family groupings will only grow. One question that may arise is how nonbiological children, for instance those created with donated sperm, will fare in these situations. Social psychology professor Susan Golombok, at City University in London, studies this phenomenon and explores how the distinction between biological and social parenting roles may influence family dynamics.[89] Her work focuses on children born by sperm donation and the worry that they may be at risk of feeling alienated from their social family.[90] Interestingly, her research shows that there is little effect, either negative or positive, for children born by reproductive technology because they are as likely to be content or to be alienated from their parents as the rest of their peer group.[91] Perhaps this is not so surprising as such "social parenting" has always been the case with remarriage after the death of one partner and with adoption.

All of the evidence presented here points to a coming explosion in family diversity. There has always been variation in human relationships and family structures, but the possible combinations are set to mushroom owing to both longer lives and extended fertility. Of course, paying for all this family activity will be a big concern for many. In the next chapter, we will address questions of finances and work in a one-hundred-plus world.

CHAPTER 6

The Financial Implications of Longevity

VIRGINIA RASKIN IS a star real estate agent in Sacramento, California, selling million-dollar homes, taking calls from clients at all hours, and processing piles of paperwork. She is what many would call a "go-getter," and in 2008 the local newspaper lauded her for "racking up sales in a down market." You might expect a person with such high energy to be middle-aged or younger, but the surprising facts about Raskin are that she's over ninety years old and this is her second career, following a career in nursing.[1] Such stories make the news because most of us hope, either secretly or otherwise, that we will also be full of energy in our older years. Fortunately, because of advances in science and technology, we are marching toward a world where there will be more people like Virginia Raskin and fewer people retiring to nursing homes in their nineties.

Money makes the world go round, and living longer means both making and spending money longer. This begs the question, then, if the average person could expect to live a healthy 150 years, how would that change the economy? Or put a slightly different way, how would extending our *economically active* life span alter our financial world? There are many elements that define an individual's economic life, including education, experience, ambition, effort, savings, and retirement plans. A country's accumulated human capital and wealth are generated from its citizens' individual choices regarding these elements. This chapter will consider the changes that longer and healthier lives will create in each of these important areas.

THE VALUE OF TIME

Time-use scholars Dr. John P. Robinson and Dr. Geoffrey Godbey note that, although leisure time has increased, regular surveys over the last thirty years have shown that American adults feel rushed either all the time or some of the time.[2] Perhaps surprisingly, even with the graying of the nation and the number of retirees increasing, this pattern hasn't changed during all these years. For example, in 1971 73 percent of all Americans reported feeling either "always" or "sometimes rushed."[3] In 2005 the numbers were similar, with 76 percent saying they were "always" or "sometimes" rushed.[4] This feeling of time pressure results in humorous articles with titles like "Too Busy to Notice You're Too Busy." On a more serious level, however, our feelings of busyness are inherently linked with both economic growth and how much time we have. These two factors also happen to be significantly affected by life span.

In 1965 Nobel laureate Gary Becker wrote a paper titled "A Theory of the Allocation of Time," discussing how time constitutes a significant part of the true cost of anything. The insight of the paper suggests that the cost of time *changes* based on the nature of a commodity and the length of time under consideration. For instance, the cost of time is less for activities like sleeping and eating as compared with going to the theater because sleeping and eating contribute to a person's productive effort. That is, people can't really do anything else if they are weak from sleep or food deprivation. In addition, he argued that "the cost of time is often less on weekends and in the evenings because many firms are closed then."[5] The idea that the cost of time changes depending on circumstances could have great implications for a world in which people gained more time, a world where humans expanded their life expectancy by a factor of two.

Becker wasn't the only one to realize that the price of time changes. In an insightful little book titled *The Harried Leisure Class*, Swedish economist Staffan Linder explains why, even with the great economic growth Western nations have experienced, individuals don't seem to be more relaxed. In fact, as the preceding polling data attest, most of us seem rather harried. It turns out that economic growth also changes how we spend our time. As wages go up (and time stays fixed), it becomes more expensive to do things away from work. Consuming things like movies or books takes time that we might have otherwise spent working, so increasing wages makes our nonwork time more expensive.[6]

Both Becker and Linder logically assumed fixed amounts of time. There are only 24 hours in a day, after all, and life expectancy in 1965 was about 70 years.[7] Out of 24 hours, if we assume 8 are spent sleeping, that means only 16 are left for work and nonwork activities. So if we multiply 16 by 365 days in a year by 70 years, that means the average person in 1965 had 408,800 hours during his life in which to do things. But what if one of the variables in the equation changes? What if the average life expectancy increases? If average life expectancy increased to 150, the number of hours that a person would have to spend would equal 876,000 hours. That is a big increase in the amount of time and therefore may have an impact on the value of time and thus on how harried people feel. Because an increase in economic growth can change how time is valued, we will also need to examine the extent to which economic growth might change as a result of greater longevity.

THE RELATIONSHIP
BETWEEN HEALTH AND WEALTH

Economist Julian Simon was famous for arguing that "the ultimate resource is people—especially skilled, spirited, and hopeful *young people* endowed with liberty—who will exert their wills and imaginations for their own benefit, and so inevitably they will benefit the rest of us as well" (my italics).[8] One of the reasons for this emphasis on young people is that they are generally *healthy* and have the energy to pick up big projects and run with them. They are also often doing things for the first time, which potentially gives them a different perspective from those who have been in the field for a while.

So how will longer health spans change our stock of human capital? First, and perhaps most importantly, healthy directly implies better and more productive human capital. This is perhaps an obvious conclusion, but it wasn't until relatively recently that researchers began investigating whether health actually creates wealth.

For many years it's been clear that there is a positive correlation between health and wealth, but it was most commonly thought that wealth creates health. Even though it is certainly true that the rich can afford to take better care of themselves, we now know that health also begets wealth. Put another way, poor health causes a decline in productivity for the simple reason that it's very difficult to work effectively when you're in ill health, thereby increasing your chances of falling into poverty.

In their paper titled "The Health and Wealth of Nations," Harvard economist David Bloom and Queen's University economist David Canning explain that, based on the available research, if there are "two countries that are identical in all respects, except that one has a 5 year advantage in life expectancy," then the "real income per capita in the healthier country will grow 0.3–0.5% per year faster than in its less healthy counterpart."[9] Although these percentages might look small, they are actually quite significant, especially when we consider that between 1965 and 1990 countries experienced an average per capita income growth of 2 percent per year. When countries only have an average growth of that amount, an advantage of 0.5 percent is quite the boost.

Now, those numbers are based on only a five-year longevity advantage. What if a country had a ten-, twenty-, or thirty-year advantage? The growth might not continue on a linear basis, but if the general rule holds—a jump in life expectancy causes an increase in economic growth per capita—then having a longer-lived population would facilitate enormous differences in economic prosperity.[10] This helps to explain why there is a movement among some academics and activists to urge Congress to spend more on antiaging research in order to create what they call a "longevity dividend."[11] For instance, public health professor S. Jay Olshansky argues that slowing aging by only three to seven years would "simultaneously postpone all fatal and nonfatal disabling diseases, produce gains in health and longevity equivalent to cures for major fatal diseases, and create scientific, medical, and economic windfalls for future generations that would be roughly equivalent in impact to the discovery of antibiotics in the 20th century."[12] His enthusiasm is justified, given that economists have demonstrated that improvements in health were a major contributor to well-being over the course of the twentieth century.

In 2006 University of Chicago economists Kevin Murphy and Robert Topel painstakingly calculated that for Americans, "gains in life expectancy over the century were worth over $1.2 million per person to the current population."[13] They also found that "from 1970 to 2000, gains in life expectancy added about $3.2 trillion *per year* to national wealth."[14] These enormous numbers represent a spectacular accomplishment in terms of benefits. Indeed, it could be said that longevity gains are really the best thing humans have ever accomplished. This explosion of wealth creation contributes a significant amount to the well-being of Americans, but they are not the only ones gaining from longer lives.

Around the world researchers have shown that longevity gains have caused an increase in economic welfare across the board and the countries with the biggest gains have been the less-developed nations.[15] For example, a study published by the National Bureau of Economic Research showed that for the time period between 1965 and 1995 the welfare gains resulting from longevity were 27 percent of gross domestic product (GDP) for Mexicans and only 5 percent for Americans born the same year. Of course, developing countries are starting from a lower GDP to begin with, so the raw numbers are larger for America, but the point is that longevity is helping people in countries everywhere and the percentage gains are bigger in the countries that are starting from a lower point. Economist Gary Becker, a coauthor of the paper, comments that "the picture of world inequality looks a bit less bleak when you take a broader economic view that accounts for the rise in life expectancy in poor countries."[16] That is, comparing countries only on per capita GDP does not take into account the full economic benefits enjoyed by a longer-living person. Benefits aside from GDP include leisure time and what economists call "nontraded goods." When a family grows its own vegetables and eats them, family members are enjoying nontraded goods. As indicated in Figure 6.1, Venezuela, El Salvador, and Egypt have been the biggest beneficiaries of longevity on a percentage basis.

One other thing that may also make world inequality seem a bit less bleak, as Becker puts it, is the fact that much of the cost of these welfare gains are borne by developed countries, which disproportionately pay more for creating and developing the technologies that bring about the gains in longevity.

THE ROLE OF EDUCATION

Clearly, longer-lived individuals add to the economic welfare of any country by virtue of being around longer to work, but living longer also allows for more time to get educated. This is important because education increases the *quality* of human capital, which matters quite a bit when it comes to the financial well-being of both individuals and nations.[17] Figure 6.2 contains data from the U.S. Department of Labor showing how education pays off on a personal level, benefiting the individual in terms of higher wages and lower unemployment.

These results on the individual level also track on the national and international levels. If one person can make a lot more money by

FIGURE 6.1

Share of Welfare Improvements Due to Longevity Gains

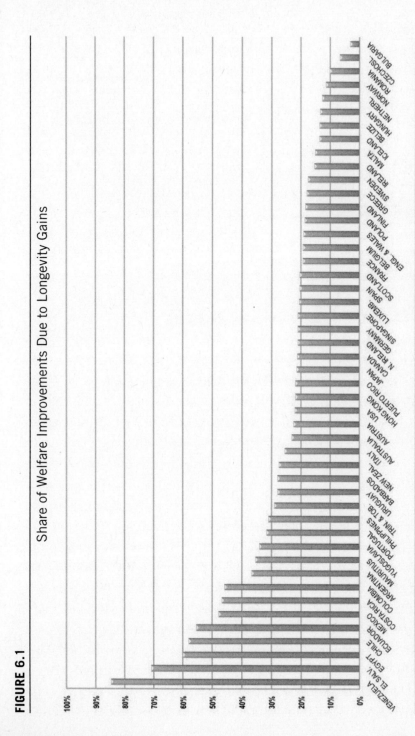

SOURCE: Based on Gary Becker, Tomas J. Philipson, and Rodrigo R. Soares, "The Quantity and Quality of Life and the Evolution of World Inequality," Paper no. 9765 (Cambridge, MA: National Bureau of Economic Research, June 2003).

FIGURE 6.2

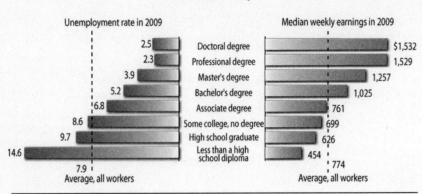

Education Pays

SOURCE: U.S. Department of Labor, Bureau of Labor Statistics, Current Population Survey, 2009, www.bls.gov/emp/ep_chart_001.htm.

obtaining a higher education, then just imagine what can happen when a large group of people collectively increase their education. In a paper funded by the National Science Foundation, economists Rodolfo Manuelli and Ananth Seshadri from the University of Wisconsin–Madison demonstrate that a good deal of the differences in the economic output of countries is due to differences in human capital, a large portion of which is formed through education.

"To be precise," they write, "the typical individual in a poor country not only chooses to acquire fewer years of schooling, he also acquires less human capital per year of schooling."[18] The finding that education and the quality of that education matter in terms of economic output is not surprising and is one of the reasons that a high-performing school system is important for economic growth.

Individuals make choices on how much education to acquire based on the future value of that educational investment compared to their next-best alternatives. This means that when people make the decision to go to school, they compare their forgone earnings during school with the extra income they expect to get after they've completed the schooling. Education levels rise when people live longer because the future value of education rises. That is, if an individual works for only forty years following higher education, he gets forty years of higher wages; but if he works for seventy years, he gets seventy years at a higher wage—a significant difference in wealth. Indeed, throughout history longer lives are correlated with greater education.

In the United States in 1900 only 10 percent of teenagers were enrolled in high school; in 1940, 70 percent of teenagers were enrolled in high school; and in 2000, 95 percent of teenagers were enrolled in high school.[19] But it is not just quantity of education that matters; quality is important, too. We might ask, then, if longer lives will drive demand for higher-quality educational programs. In a longer-lived and interconnected world, global competition will increase and quality education will be paramount to success. Of course, there is no guarantee that any individual country will automatically create a better system, but the pressure to do so will certainly rise. Perhaps one sign of this growing pressure was the production of the 2010 documentary film *Waiting for Superman*, in which Academy Award–winning director Davis Guggenheim highlighted problems with education in America, including restrictive policies on firing teachers, a touchy subject that few are willing to take on.[20] And while fixing a failed system is of paramount importance, it may also be worth considering how educational needs might change as longevity extends.

In his book *Five Minds for the Future*, Harvard psychology and education professor Howard Gardner argues that there are five traits that need cultivation in order to create a successful economy going forward.[21] These are discipline, the ability to synthesize data, creativity, respectfulness, and ethics—all aspects that are key in a global economy with many diverse cultures. Following from this, we can see that in a world of longer health spans, such characteristics will also be highly valued because there will be the additional issue of intergenerational management. Already, older boomer generation managers complain about not understanding new employees from Generation Y (born after 1980). According to Jordan Kaplan, an associate managerial science professor at Long Island University–Brooklyn, Generation Y has "grown up questioning their parents, and now they're questioning their employers. They don't know how to shut up, which is great, but that's aggravating to the 50-year-old manager who says, 'Do it and do it now.'"[22] Such generational divides have always existed—recall, for instance, the generation that wouldn't trust anyone over thirty—but in a longer-lived world there will be more generations, which creates increased opportunities for misunderstandings or tension. Therefore, the transition to a longer-lived society will require a higher degree of cooperation between people, young and old, who differ widely in their group cultures and language.

How is the face of the classroom changed by these forces? Data from Australian universities show that enrollment statistics are becoming increasingly age-integrated and are now widely defined as lifelong.[23] Even though empirically these findings suggest that learning is trending toward more investment throughout life, the findings do not support the idea that there will be a decreasing amount of intensive training periods at the beginning of life. In fact, as implied earlier, because people will have longer health spans, there will likely be an increase in the amount of time they spend in training at the beginning of their lives as well as throughout their lives. This begs the question of whether educational delivery will change as our lives lengthen and we become more technologically sophisticated.

Education likely will expand to offer more personalized instruction. In a recent book titled *Disrupting Class*, Clayton Christensen and his coauthors make a persuasive case that the future of education will become more tailored to individuals' learning styles and levels. Whereas one student might learn best from rote memorization, another might be better off learning through an interactive game format or virtual reality system. Christensen sees better computers and software as the platform for providing this individualized training. Computer-based learning, he says, "will keep improving, as all successful disruptions do. It will become more enjoyable and take full advantage of the online medium by layering in enhanced video, audio, and interactive elements."[24] As virtual reality experiences become possible, education will move to a whole new level. A day may well come when an executive comes home from work, has dinner, and then spends an hour engaged in her virtual learning environment instead of watching TV. This will happen partly because the learning experience will be more enjoyable and partly because continual learning will be required to stay competitive.

EXTREME EXPERIENCE

In September 2008 *BusinessWeek* magazine published a story featuring twenty-five influential business leaders who also happened to be over the age of seventy-five. The list included Osamu Suzuki, who at seventy-eight "still call[ed] the shots" at Suzuki Motor; Harold Burson, who at eighty-seven still offered cutting-edge advice to clients at public-relations firm Burson-Marsteller; and Sumner Redstone, who at eighty-five was chairman of CBS and Viacom.[25] As the magazine noted, these men were not average CEOs and chairmen, yet the unspoken premise was that one day they could be as more and more business leaders remain in the workforce for longer periods of time.

Life expectancy has grown linearly at an average rate of 3 months per year (2.5 years per decade) for women and 2.5 months per year (2 years per decade) for men and, as argued in Chapter 2, is about to grow much more.[26] When that happens, and health span is extended, it will be possible to have 130-year-olds and over at the helm of companies. What advantages will come with greater numbers of healthy, older workers?

Aside from historical knowledge and large rolodexes, older workers tend to be more patient. In 2006 researchers from Harvard showed that patience increases across the life span.[27] They showed that with age people tend to stop discounting the future and learn to become more future oriented (until, of course, they reach the point where they think they have no future left). Once life expectancy significantly expands, there should be an increased number of workers who are educated, experienced, and more patient. This patience may allow for steadfastness in the accomplishment of goals, more harmony in personal relationships, and clearer foresight when approaching problems. Such mature behavior will allow for an increased ability to put off present pleasure for future gains and, we can hope, cultivate leaders who deal reasonably and fairly with generations other than their own. But even with these benefits, one question that immediately comes to mind is the impact on the job market. How can younger individuals hope to move up the ladder when those at the top don't retire when they reach sixty-five, seventy-five, eighty-five, or more?

There are different ways to approach this question, the first of which is to acknowledge that just because these leaders have experience doesn't necessarily mean that they will always win in the marketplace. Make no mistake: experience is an important part of human capital, but it is not the sum. Other attributes, such as creativity, motivation, effort, flexibility, intelligence, and talent, come into play as well. Indeed, the *BusinessWeek* story pointed out that a "calculation shows that most of the seniors on our list who run public companies failed to beat their respective indexes over the past five years."[28] Experience was clearly an asset, but it didn't mean that these select and very experienced executives were able to beat the stock market.

Another way to look at the question of whether older workers will create barriers to younger people seeking higher positions is to consider what kinds of businesses are likely to employ people. In the United States, about half of all workers are employed by small businesses. As long as starting a business remains relatively easy, small businesses, which can turn into big businesses, are one avenue for young people looking to build experience. And in a world where technology will continue to help level playing fields, businesses that shun smart, young people will face competitive disadvantages. There are many examples of young people starting small companies that grew into larger, very successful companies. For example, Steve Jobs and Steve Wozniak started Apple in their early twenties—the same age as Bill Gates and Paul Allen when they started Microsoft—and Sergey Brin and Larry Page launched Google in their mid-twenties.

GOING LONG ON AMBITION

The degree to which longevity will change the economic order also depends somewhat on how much of an effect an increased health span has on the conditions of human ambition. A strong source of motivation, ambition affects individuals and societies on a large scale. Longer health spans mean that individuals no longer have to curtail life plans so that they accomplish only what can be accomplished in the formerly expected life span of around 80 years. That is, an individual's aspirations will no longer be limited to achieving what he expects to achieve in less than 100 years. For instance, when Donald Boudreaux, former chairman of the Department of Economics at George Mason University, was asked about his current life expectancy and career plans, the over-50-year-old said, "I won't [have time to do work that will] win a Nobel Prize, so I am focusing on communicating economics to the public."[29] But what if Dr. Boudreaux had more time? He might still not win a Nobel Prize, but he might try new projects that he thought could lead him there, and that activity would be good for society. Consider that in the future an equivalent human to the Greek scientist Archimedes could walk the earth for 150 years, making so many contributions to society that for at least the initial social acclimation to increased longevity, he might seem godlike. Of course, once society became acclimatized to longer working years, Archimedes would still be significant, but our sense of his accomplishments would be qualified by our recognition that he didn't have that long a life.

It might be tempting here to argue that longer lives could harm ambition because they would allow more time to procrastinate. Perhaps some will look at increased longevity that way, but because longer lives do not mean immortal lives, individuals will know that their time is limited and that their lives could come to an end at any moment through an accident or other misfortune. This knowledge should tilt things in favor of enhanced ambition, and for some that will mean having multiple careers. Today, if someone dreams of being both a lawyer and a doctor, it is unlikely that she will do both. However, in a world with longer health spans, a person could very well have two distinct careers that each require a significant amount of education.

There have always been certain individuals who work their whole lives and never retire. They do so not because they need money, but because they are ambitious and enjoy building wealth, power, and knowledge. In a world where some of these individuals live to be 150 years old, the corporate empires they build could be bigger than anything we've ever seen. But what about the opposite argument that only the young are ambitious and creative? It's true that there are certain fields, like mathematics, professional athletics, and heavy manual labor, where the best performers peak early and don't seem to be able to sustain their productivity. The reason for the early peak in math is unclear, but when it comes to sports and labor, the problem is a breakdown in the body. In contrast, many other fields, such as literature, economics, philosophy, musical composition, painting, leadership, and invention, spur careers in which people continue to contribute throughout life or even peak at later ages. For instance, Leonardo da Vinci was fifty-one when he started painting the Mona Lisa and Wilhelm Conrad Röntgen was fifty when he discovered the X-ray.[30] Benjamin Franklin was forty-six when he did his famous kite experiment verifying the nature of electricity, but he didn't stop there. He was fifty-five when he invented the glass harmonica and seventy-eight when he invented bifocals.[31] If Franklin had had the opportunity to live longer in a healthier state, what else would he have contributed to society? As U.S. Court of Appeals judge Richard Posner argues, the fact that invention seems to be a "late peak" field "should allay concerns that the aging of the population threatens to reduce the rate of inventive activity, and with it the economic growth that is due to that activity."[32]

Of course, not everyone is excited about more years to work. "Let's face it," says Chris Hackler, director of medical humanities at the University of Arkansas, "most people's jobs aren't all that fascinating."[33] That is true, but with longer life expectancies, people would have the opportunity to retrain to do something more appealing to them, and the amount of time away from work, in the total calculation, would also jump. Let's compare the life expectancy of someone born in 1900, around 48 years, to both the current average of around 80 years and a future potential of 150 years. Someone with a 48-year run would get to enjoy only 2,496 weekends and 17,520 evenings during which he might go to concerts or enjoy time with family. In contrast, living to 80 years allows for 4,160 weekends and 29,200 evenings, and living to 150 means 7,800 available weekends and 54,750 evenings (see Figure 6.3).

Savvy readers will point out that the figure assumes a constant ratio of workdays to weekends, but if new technologies or increased productivity result in more leisure time, as they have in the past, then there may be even more time away from work to focus on personal

FIGURE 6.3

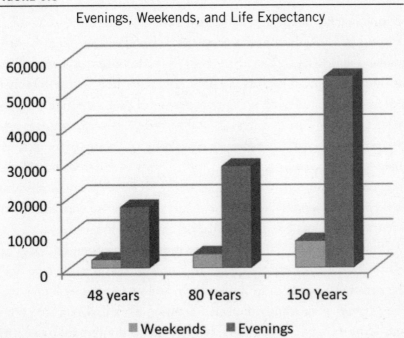

Evenings, Weekends, and Life Expectancy

■ Weekends ■ Evenings

interests. How do changes in technology or productivity result in more free time? Consider an example involving a common home appliance: the dishwasher. Those without dishwashers might spend forty-five minutes each night cleaning up after dinner, whereas those with a dishwasher might clean for five minutes. The forty-minute gain could be used to go running, watch TV, or surf the Internet.

THE PERSISTENCE OF WORK
AND A REDEFINITION OF RETIREMENT

Given that leisure time grows when workers become more efficient through technology and improved skills, will a combination of accelerating technology and enhanced human capital eventually make work a tiny part of our lives? The answer depends on a number of factors, including how much our extra years and corresponding wealth creation affect our preferences for trading between work and leisure activities. For years leisure experts and futurists have been predicting that as the economy grows, work will start to fade away. Yet as of this writing, work was still a significant part of our daily lives. According to the U.S. Bureau of Labor Statistics, individuals between twenty-five and fifty-four worked an average of 8.7 hours a day and had 2.6 hours for leisure and sports.[34] That's not to say that leisure time has not increased along with economic growth and life expectancy. As already noted, it has. But work is still of paramount importance, and when we do engage in leisure, such as skiing and going to movies, we make ourselves busy—sometimes to the point of underestimating our free time. Perhaps it is this circumstance that led time-use scholars Robinson and Godbey to comment that "workers are working somewhat shorter hours but estimate they are working longer."[35]

It should also be noted that many workers now spend more time *at work* doing leisure activities such as surfing the Internet, conducting personal business, running errands, and socializing with coworkers. This growing interconnection between work and personal time may help to explain why some workers today are not interested in retiring. For instance, eighty-four-year-old Jean Hines of St. Louis, Missouri, says that she continues her job at an airplane parts manufacturing plant because she "can't just sit at home." The work seems to give her more purpose than she might have otherwise.[36]

A more convincing reason for the persistence of work, despite increased wealth, is capital accumulation. As workers' wages increase, they will find it difficult or perhaps even undesirable to have too much leisure time *at any given time* for fear of missing out on additional capital and extra experience in the workforce. This will likely mean a rejection of opportunities to take off large chunks of time to golf, travel the world, or retire early.

It's already common knowledge that most of us don't expect a retirement that starts at 65. The social security system cannot afford it even now, and in a longevity-enhanced society going out to the pasture to rest at 65 gets boring for the person living to 150.[37] Instead, many will use additional life years for secondary and tertiary life goals. For example, those who struggled between a career path in medicine or starting their own business could choose both dreams, and "retirement" might be redefined to mean the expensive chunk of time that someone takes out of regular working life in order to train extensively for a new career. A person could spend thirty years in the business world, thirty years as a doctor, and an additional twenty-five years accumulating human capital through education. Because of the ability to achieve secondary and tertiary life goals, people may put off retirement until serious disability occurs, and work hours will decline only as a result of health decreases in the latter half of a 150-year life span. Such a shift could be seen as a throwback to agrarian societies, where retirement didn't really exist. Back then people worked the fields until they just couldn't anymore. The difference, of course, is that in the future people will be much wealthier than were those in agrarian societies and will likely not be doing manual labor. Indeed, retirement itself is a relatively new concept that was only officially made into American law after President Franklin D. Roosevelt proposed the Social Security Act of 1935.[38]

An alternative to this view is that longer lives may spur an even greater movement toward part-time and flex-time work because older individuals will not want to leave the workforce but will not wish to put in full days either. It's also possible that there will be those who do want a more traditional retirement at the end of life, and those are the people most likely to be good at saving. Whichever way it goes, there clearly will be more opportunity for diversity in economic choices.

SAVINGS AND INVESTMENT

No matter how the balance between work and retirement is resolved, there will remain a period of human life when individual income will be dependent on capital already accumulated by the individual or provided by society as a whole. One interesting finding is that within the United States many who already live to around one hundred have both planned financially for their retirement and continued to accumulate capital postretirement.[39] A study conducted by Thomas Perls, assistant professor at Harvard Medical School, and his colleague Lara Terry showed that their sample of centenarians "had lived 30 years beyond what they expected to live, and they still had a little extra."[40]

However, not everyone is so good at planning, and evidence from across the Organisation for Economic Co-operation and Development (OECD) suggests that people tend to feel they have saved too little for their retirement.[41] Why is this the case, and how will longer lives change an individual's propensity to save? This is a complicated question, and economists disagree on both the proper level of saving and how to get people to save more. Irving Fisher, who was arguably America's first celebrity economist, maintained that there are six personal characteristics that influence savings. They are short- or longsightedness, level of self-control, habits of thrift, expectation of length of life, desire to leave money after death, and susceptibility to social pressure to spend, such as the idea of keeping up with the Joneses.[42] Obviously, this is a large basket of traits, but at least three of Fisher's six characteristics may be influenced by longer lives. These are the degree of short/longsightedness, the expectation of length of life, and the desire to leave money after death.

Once health spans expand and average life expectancy reaches 150 years, expectations about length of life will grow. Longer lives mean that there is a longer period of time to be around, which may increase each individual's amount of uncertainty. Accidents, epidemics, and other miseries will not disappear even when science is better able to repair the human body.[43] Greater uncertainty typically generates higher savings, as people begin to put money away just in case things don't work out as planned. Of course, many things can affect the population's degree of certainty. For instance, governments that promise new social benefits may help reduce uncertainty and affect the savings rate. At the moment, however, social security in the United States is troubled, and a longer life should prompt greater savings, not only because of increased uncertainty, but also because there will be more time to save.

The other two characteristics—degree of short- or longsightedness and desire to leave money after death—are even more difficult to use as predictors, but there are some things we might say about how they could affect savings. A theory called the life cycle hypothesis says that the time horizons individuals use to plan are equal to life expectancy, but various scholars have shown that time horizons vary for different decision areas and different people.[44] This has led Swedish economic psychologist Karl-Erik Warneryd to conclude that there is no hard-and-fast rule when it comes to people's time horizons.[45] Yet planning for retirement requires long-term thinking.

Both economists and psychologists maintain that the vividness of a future image is important in determining whether people follow through with savings or not. Put another way, it is easy to imagine how that new pair of shoes will look on you tomorrow if you buy them today, but it is harder to imagine how saving now will allow you to go back to school while maintaining the same standard of living in ten years. It could be argued that in a world where people are increasingly living longer, it will be easier to imagine living a very long time because people actually living longer will be there to see. Indeed, one day banks and other financial institutions might take an even greater interest in advertising to consumers about how saving now will create many more opportunities later.[46] This type of advertising and potential cultural shift in thinking about the future may influence Fisher's category of short- versus longsightedness. If individuals can see other people living their dreams through savings, as well as being told about it through various media outlets, longer lives may increase people's propensity toward longsightedness. One already-developed technology that might make such advocacy easier is automated financial goal planning software. For instance, Mint, an online personal finance tool that was bought by Intuit, helps users find personalized ways to save money and could one day better help users track and reach long-term financial goals. Such personalized help from computer programs is only the beginning of where banks can make inroads with a population that is about to live longer and may not be saving enough for current life expectancies.

The last of Fisher's characteristics that could be influenced by longer lives is bequests, or the desire to leave money for loved ones or for society in general after death. Understandably, a common conclusion on the future of bequests is that older people are now spending most of the money that otherwise would have been left as an inheritance in times gone by. Today, with increased health care costs at the end of life, and with many older people healthy enough to spend their time traveling and shopping, many children expect to see their inheritance shrink or disappear altogether. Indeed, according to a 2010 study by scholars at the Center for Retirement Research at Boston College, the median inheritance that Boomers can expect is $64,000, slightly more than the cost for one year at a private college.[47] However, that is the situation today. It could continue, but other factors, such as potentially less expensive health care (we will discuss this in a moment) and compound interest combined with larger family structures, could come into play and shift motivations.

There will always be a certain percentage of the population that doesn't save, but longer lives could tilt the scales in favor of increasing, not decreasing, personal savings. At this point, we should also note that any savings invested at a younger age would be earning interest over a longer period of time than ever before. Because compounding works by adding accumulated interest back to the principal, interest is continually earned on whatever principal there was plus the interest that the individual has already made. This means that money grows at a much faster rate when saved in this manner than if stuffed in the mattress. Indeed, compounding works so well that Albert Einstein called it the "eighth wonder of the world." For example, if a person saved $100,000 at age 30, the value at age 65 would be $551,602 and the value at age 130 would be $13,150,126 (assuming, for simplicity, compound interest of 5 percent and no additional savings). This can be contrasted with a person who saves the same amount under the same conditions but doesn't begin until age 50. That person would have only $207,893 at age 65 and $4,956,144 at age 130.

Clearly, older people who started saving at a younger age will bene-fit the most from compound interest, and because people in a longer-lived world could be incentivized to save more, that would mean that older people would have more money than they do today. Of course, large sums of money don't negate the fact that there will be costs. Health care costs are usually highest near the end of life, and large amounts are often spent trying to fight the inevitable. Indeed, as *New York Times* writer Bob Morris has pointed out, he and many others worry that health costs will consume what they eventually receive from their parents.

"Much as I hate to admit it," Morris writes, "there were plenty of moments during the last year when I was consumed with an invis-ible ledger in my brain: my inheritance versus [my father's] health costs. Fifteen hundred dollars a week on this. Six thousand a month on that. It could all add up to leaving nothing."[48] Will this trend continue? Will all the new technologies just wind up adding more and more expenses at the end of life that will eat up even the greater savings that people with radically extended lives will accumulate? Perhaps, but not necessarily. Consider that when doctors are able to grow a new heart for a patient out of her own tissue, taking drugs to fix symptoms of a sick heart will no longer be necessary and there will be fewer trips to the emergency room afterward, saving money. Likewise, if technology leads to a greater compression of morbidity, people can expect to be healthy for longer, with shorter periods of sickness that call for expensive techniques to keep them alive.

MORE OR LESS HARRIED?

One of the questions raised at the beginning of this chapter was whether individuals will feel less "harried" as they gain more time owing to greater longevity. Factors that influence the answer to this question include amount of time gained, levels of economic growth, and preferences in the tradeoff between money (productivity) and leisure. Given that the amount of time each individual possesses over a life will expand, but productivity will as well, the likely outcome for a country like the United States that highly values productivity is that people will remain harried. Talk show hosts, women's magazines, and celebrity trainers can rest assured that there will always be a large market of people interested in hearing about Dr. Oz's "maximize your time workout." Greater wealth generation will give individuals more resources with which to occupy their increased time (leisure and otherwise), and they will likely fill up their calendars as they do today. The upside, however, is that more time and greater wealth translate into more experiences that can contribute to individual growth and self-actualization. The possibilities are endless.

With more weekends in a person's life, there can be more short getaways to wine country or more chances to see a favorite team play soccer. For those who like to shop, the combination of greater time and wealth is obvious. There will also be new possibilities such as space travel or real-seeming virtual reality worlds. And additional experiences will certainly be created through formal education, which can be expected to increase over the life span because continual learning will be required even more than it is today to stay competitive in the marketplace.

Taking time off work to get reeducated might become the new definition of retirement. When people can stay healthy and vibrant for longer periods and reduce their disability time before death, retirement as we know it today won't be the standard option. Diversity of options will increase, and individuals will not look forward to traditional retirement, but will instead look forward to taking time off to start a new career or pursue other life interests.

Death will still be a fact of life in a longer-lived world, and ambition will not disappear. Indeed, longer life spans give the superambitious even more time to create and grow their empires. Jack Welch is no longer CEO of General Electric, but he still enjoys giving advice through his Web site, magazine columns, and an MBA program he started in 2009—just imagine what he would do if he thought he had an extra fifty healthy years ahead of him.[49]

Having so many vibrant older people around poses a potential problem for the job prospects of younger people, but it is not an insurmountable issue. Society has an interest in intergenerational harmony, and corporations will have limits on how much they are willing to pay for experience. Younger people, who will be paid less, may be a better bargain for employers who are looking to streamline their business costs. That said, there will be intergenerational tensions simply because of cultural differences. Any boomer who has tried to manage someone from generation Y knows that even now the challenges can be great.

National savings rates were quite low between 2005 and 2007, but they have recently gone up and longer lives may help drive that upward trend. That is, increased uncertainly associated with longer lives could spur more people to get serious about saving. New technologies like online financial management tools can help individuals learn to better manage their funds. For those who are diligent, compound interest will have an even bigger impact on their bottom line, as more time means greater wealth-generation opportunities.

That, then, is the story of wealth and worldly goods in a time of longer health spans. It's only fair next to turn to our souls and those who purport to care for them.

CHAPTER 7

The Afterlife Versus a Longer Life

Religion in the Age of Longevity

The last enemy that shall be destroyed is death.
—1 CORINTHIANS 15:26

WOODY ALLEN ONCE joked, "I don't want to achieve immortality through my work; I want to achieve it through not dying." His statement effectively makes light of humanity's collective anxiety over death, an issue that can be traced back to the very beginning of human culture.[1] From East to West, every religion promises transcendence to some form of an afterlife, whether it is heaven, hell, Jannah, Jahannam, nirvana, or moksa. Life after death is one of the most compelling aspects of religious belief, and some scholars, such as Pulitzer Prize–winning cultural anthropologist Ernest Becker, have suggested that without death, religion would not exist.[2] The quest to obtain everlasting life is responsible for many projects throughout history, but the main question this chapter addresses is, what happens to this drive and the organizations that support it, such as churches and mosques, in a world where humans move further away from death? Put another way, if science and technology can help us live much longer lives, will we begin to imagine immorality here on earth, and if so, will that affect our motivation to connect with God?

A GLIMPSE OF IMMORTALITY

In 2006 60 *Minutes* aired a program titled "The Quest for Immortality" in which the venerated media institution opened with these sentences: "How's this for an offer you can't refuse: how would you like to live say, 400 or 500 years, or even more and all of them in perfect health? . . . There are those who say it is well within the realm of possibility."[3] In 2008 *The Economist* published an article with similar sentiments, titled "How to Live Forever: Abolishing Ageing."[4] If such claims have already reached levels like these based on *predicted* trajectories of how science will affect life expectancies, just imagine the level of discussion once the science *actually* starts paying off. The conversations will no longer be about how long we can live, but about how we can stave off death forever. Once the discussion hits that point, religion could be in trouble because a big part of its appeal is the promise of immortality in the afterlife. If individuals can achieve immortality here on earth, why bother with another realm?

Scholars of religion have already started discussions about this quandary. In the seminal compilation on the topic, *Religion and the Implications of Radical Life Extension*, edited by religious studies professors Derek Maher and Calvin Mercer, Rabbi Elliot N. Dorff predicts that longer lives will make religious messages weaker. "The longer we think we have until we die," Rabbi Dorff cautions, "the less likely it is that the reality of death will affect our lives. Just as it is very difficult to convince people in their teens and twenties that they need to take their mortality into account, a prolonged life will likely strengthen and lengthen our pursuit of fame and fortune."[5] Jain scholar and professor of religious studies Sherry E. Fohr agrees. "Fear of harmful karma and therefore bad rebirths is a significant motivating factor for many Jains. Without death, this motivation would cease to exist, and this could lead to a decrease in the number of Jains who are religious."[6]

Clearly, life extension is going to put one of the big selling points of religion at risk, but does that mean that religion will completely lose its appeal? Not a chance, argues theology and ethics professor Ronald

Cole-Turner. He maintains that the difference between life extension on earth and the afterlife is too significant. "Christianity offers life, not by making us immortal, but by making us new. The essential feature of that transformation is not longevity but a renewed relationship with God."[7] In fact, Cole-Turner argues that to extend life without attending to the soul would be hell on earth. In the end, he says, "it is not our bodies or our metabolism or our telomeres that most need fixing. It is the whole person that needs to be changed, the whole self, in particular the tendency to turn inward, away from others and away from God."[8] Chapman University economist Lawrence Iannaccone studies the economics of religion and agrees that many may see it this way, but he puts the matter in slightly different terms. "Supernaturalism is the all-purpose technology," he says. "You can use it for everything. Just look at how everything people care about is covered in the religious section of bookstores."[9]

LOSING OUR RELIGION—REEXAMINED

"God is dead," proclaimed German philosopher Friedrich Nietzsche in 1882. It's a statement many have made since, yet it always seems to be premature. Before we address how more time to live could affect religious practices and beliefs, we need to consider a sometimes-popular assumption about the relationship between progress and religion. In the 1960s scholars led by Peter Berger, author of *The Sacred Canopy*, argued that as society advanced and became more modern, religion would invariably fade. "Our underlying argument was that secularization and modernity go hand in hand," Berger says.[10] It's a theory that seems to make sense, at least to many Westerners, because science often looks poised to find answers to things religion only begins to explain. As popular astrophysicist Carl Sagan put it, "As science advances, there seems to be less and less for God to do."[11] Such attitudes even led *The Economist* at the end of the millennium to write an "obituary" for God.[12] But although science makes important discoveries on a regular basis, the religious nature of people around the world has not withered away. Berger himself humbly admits that "I think what I and most other sociologists of religion wrote in the 1960s about secularization was a mistake."[13] Today, he says, "you cannot plausibly maintain that modernity necessarily leads to secularization: it may—and it does in certain parts of the world among certain groups of people—but not necessarily."[14] Even though the data on religiosity are notoriously complicated, most scholars in the field agree that the world has not rapidly secularized as anticipated, and some even argue that the number of religiously minded people has *grown* globally since 1970.

Dr. Todd Johnson, editor of the World Religion Database published by Brill, explains that "the world is less religious today than in 1900, but more religious since 1970 because of a resurgence of religion in post-communist countries and eastern Europe" (see Figure 7.1).[15] This complements research conducted by Harvard University political scientist Pippa Norris and University of Michigan political scientist Ronald Inglehart, who directs the World Values Survey. They write, "The world as a whole now has more people with traditional religious views than ever before—and they constitute a growing proportion of the world's population."[16] If such data weren't surprising enough, some scholars have shown that belief in an afterlife has increased in the United States, a wealthy and developed nation that has always been highly religious.[17]

Research published by the University of Chicago's Andrew M. Greeley and the University of California, Berkeley's Michael Hout demonstrates that "a greater fraction of American adults believed in life after death in the 1990s than in the 1970s."[18] Who exactly are the people that now believe in the afterlife when they didn't before? As we might expect, individuals who previously had "no religious affiliation" say they now believe in an afterlife, but, perhaps surprisingly, they are joined by both Catholics and Jews who previously weren't convinced. According to Greeley and Hout, "The percentage of Catholics believing in an afterlife rose from 67 percent to 85 percent" and "among Jews, this percentage increased from 17 percent to 74 percent."[19] How do we explain this shift?

FIGURE 7.1

Percent of World Population Belonging to Religion or No Religion

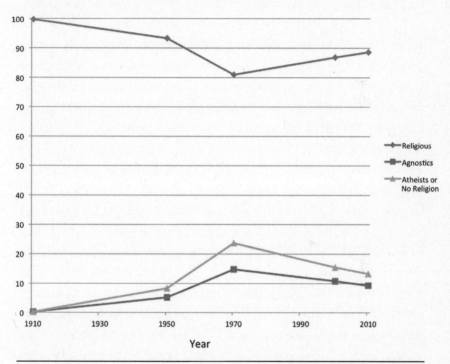

SOURCE: Based on data in Todd M. Johnson and Brian J. Grim, "International Religious Demography: An Overview of Sources and Methodology," in *The Oxford Handbook of the Economics of Religion*, ed. Rachel M. McCleary (Oxford, UK: Oxford University Press, 2011), 375.

Part of the reason, say Greeley and Hout, is owing to changes occurring within the religions, but part can also be explained by religious competition. In the United States many religions are represented and even more denominations from each religion exist and compete for members. In economic terms, we can think of churches as providing "services" and each person as a potential consumer.[20] The more competition there is, the harder each organization will try to get and retain members, thereby increasing local religious education, participation, and belief. Indeed, it seems that the more religious choice there is, the more people are inclined to be religious. This is ironic, Greeley and Hout point out, because "religious pluralism, so feared by the ardent defenders of orthodoxy, turns out to be its best guarantee."[21]

This brings us back again to the ideas of Peter Berger, who has now revised his theory of secularism and what modernity actually creates. In an interview with *The Economist*, Berger explains, "We thought that the relationship was between modernization and secularization. In fact it was between modernization and pluralism."[22] That is, as societies advance and the world becomes more globalized through new communication mediums like the Internet and wireless networks, communities become more "plural," containing more religious faiths and ideas. As noted, pluralism tends to intensify competition, which can increase converts and, as the tragic events of September 11, 2001, remind us, can also create more friction between groups when religion drives politics.

All of this is not to say that the world has not secularized to a certain degree. As Dr. Todd Johnson and his colleague Dr. Brian Grim of the Pew Foundation note, "In 1910 virtually 100 percent of the world's population was religious. By 2000 this had fallen to 87 percent."[23] Instead, what is clear is that progress, and in particular *scientific* progress, does not guarantee that societies will become less religious. Nevertheless, researchers such as Norris and Inglehart have attempted to save the secularization thesis by revising it to predict that secularization will happen when people feel "existential security," based largely on economic security.[24] For instance, in countries with generous social security nets, people feel safer because they believe they won't lack health care or housing if they lose their job. In those societies, Norris and Inglehart say, secularization is occurring and is more likely. They argue that "religiosity is systematically related at the individual level to the distribution of income groups in postindustrial societies: the poor are almost twice as religious as the rich."[25]

Even though many poor people are religious, so are many wealthy people. Consider that the $27 million Creation Museum in Kentucky was not bankrolled by poor people.[26] Indeed, as *The Economist*'s John

Micklethwait and Adrian Wooldridge argue in their book *God Is Back,* "In much of the world it is exactly the sort of upwardly mobile, educated middle classes that Marx and Weber presumed would shed such superstitions who are driving the explosion of faith."[27] The two seasoned journalists discuss their journey around the world examining the resurgence of religion. Along the way, they find middle-class Brazilian housewives who meet for exorcisms, the new bourgeoisie in Turkey and India fervently embracing religion, and young technologists in China downloading sermons and other religious material over the Internet. Stunningly, Micklethwait and Wooldridge report that there are now more Christians in China than members of the Communist Party and that one of the Chinese government's economists has published a paper arguing that Christianity is the reason for America's economic strength.[28]

Religion is an incredibly complicated topic, so there are no hard-and-fast rules to account for its strength or weakness in various areas of the world. One alternative explanation for secularism's hold in countries with strong welfare programs, such as those in Western Europe, is that government winds up filling roles traditionally carried out by religious institutions, so there are fewer opportunities for religious representatives to talk to people and convert them. Iannaccone calls this the "crowding out" effect.[29] Whatever the case, one thing is clear—religion has not disappeared and is still alive and well, even though humanity as a whole is both wealthier and healthier. So if secularism is not an obvious or guaranteed outcome as progress continues and health spans are extended, what are the options for the future of religion in a longer-lived world?

EDUCATION AND RELIGIOUS EXPERIENCE

In a 2010 television broadcast by Agence France-Presse, students from a religious school called Liberty University visit Washington's Smithsonian Museum of Natural History to view examples of Darwinian evolution. In the interview, one of the students tells the reporter that

Darwin's theory is "a fairy tale" and that "all this could have happened, but it is nothing with depth." The teachers guiding them argue with a straight face that dinosaurs died only around 5,000 years ago. Their textbook is the Bible's Old Testament.[30]

Such stories make most educated people cringe and propel atheists like Richard Dawkins to complain that such miseducation is tantamount to child abuse. It's no wonder, then, that the idea that "religious people are stupid" has taken hold in some quarters, but such blanket statements are not useful, and the reality is much more complicated, as we shall see.

In Chapter 6 we established that when health spans increase, as they did when humans boosted their life expectancy to around eighty years from an average of forty-three years, both education and experience grow as well. Because people will become more educated as they live longer, it makes sense to investigate the relationship between education and religion. That is, will more education cause people to become more or less religious, or will it have no impact at all?

The answer to this question relies upon what type of education a person is getting in the first place. In the case of a rigorous science-based education, some studies have found that "attending college as well as graduate school—and having an 'intellectual orientation'" are "significant predictors of who will reject or abandon their religion at some point in their life."[31] It is true that scientifically oriented education systems encourage students to question authority, which is probably one reason that fundamentalist religious leaders have been motivated to start their own schools or promote homeschooling. Indeed, fundamentalist religions skew the data on education and religion because their belief systems tend to have a negative effect on educational attainment in general. According to sociology professor Darren Sherkat, fundamentalist or sectarian religions can have a negative impact on education for a number of reasons and particularly for women because "in sectarian and fundamentalist religious communities young women are expected to marry early, have many children, and be primarily responsible for childcare."[32] It is also the case that "the narrowing of social networks and the restriction of information sources advocated in sectarian and fundamentalist religious groups is associated with smaller vocabularies, which can undermine academic success."[33] That being said, however, not all religions have fundamentalist elements, and it is not clear that belief in God automatically means that an individual is less intelligent or poorly educated. According to data collected by the Pew Forum on Religious and Public Life, Americans who identify as Orthodox, Unitarian, Jewish, Hindu, and Buddhist have slightly higher levels of college graduates among their members than do those who describe themselves as atheists (see Table 7.1).[34]

As many believers will be quick to point out, religion can have a positive effect on educational attainment because, as Sherkat's research shows, "religious participation and personal religiosity can help lower rates of substance abuse and limit activities that undermine college careers."[35] The social aspects of religious participation also help battle potential depression and anxiety, both of which are strongly associated with poor college performance. In these ways religion directly serves the purpose of higher education.

TABLE 7.1

College Graduates and Belief System I

Belief System	College Graduates (Percent)
Atheist	21
Buddhist	22
Hindu	26
Jewish	24
Orthodox	28
Unitarian	22
Total population (all beliefs)	16

SOURCE: Based on data in Pew Forum on Religion and Public Life, "Educational Level by Religious Tradition," U.S. Religious Landscape Survey, 2008, http://religions.pew forum.org/pdf/table-education-by-tradition.pdf.

Leading scientist Dr. Francis Collins, director of the National Institutes of Health and the former head of the Human Genome Project, is upset by the insinuation that religion leads to ignorance in science. Referring to polls showing that half of all scientists say they believe in God, Dr. Collins argues, "Either half my colleagues are enormously stupid or else the science of Darwinism is fully compatible with conventional religious beliefs—and equally compatible with atheism."[36] Dr. Collins himself was an atheist who turned religious later in life, and he makes it clear that religion is not universally opposed to science. Indeed, even the Catholic pope has agreed that evolution is a real force that permits "the development of biological diversity and complexity over very long periods of time."[37] To further drive home this point, Dr. Collins cites a survey that asked scientists if they believed in "a God that actively communicates with humankind." The percentage of respondents answering yes was the same in 1997 as it had been in 1916, indicating that advances in science hadn't caused a breakdown in belief among scientific investigators. But although some religions beat out atheism when it comes to higher education, others, such as those tending toward fundamentalism, do not. Specifically, Catholics, Protestants, Muslims, Mormons, and Jehovah's Witnesses have lower levels of college graduates compared with atheists (see Table 7.2).

So even though it appears that fundamentalism is associated with how much education a person gets, it is not clear that education causes people to become less religious. What education does is promote questioning, and such questioning can lead either to atheism or to a simple switch of religious affiliations. Looking at the issue from this perspective is more helpful and explains why the Pew Research Center also found that religious churn, or turnover, is much more common than most people realize.

According to Pew, "About half of American adults have changed religious affiliation at least once during their lives" and people can change more than once.[38] Over half of those who became unaffiliated say it is "because they think of religious people as hypocritical,

TABLE 7.2

College Graduates and Belief System II

Belief System	College Graduates (Percent)
Atheist	21
Catholic	16
Jehovah's Witnesses	6
Mormon	18
Muslim	14
Protestant	15
Total population (all beliefs)	16

SOURCE: Based on data in Pew Forum on Religion and Public Life, "Educational Level by Religious Tradition," U.S. Religious Landscape Survey, 2008, http://religions.pewforum.org/pdf/table-education-by-tradition.pdf.

judgmental or insincere, because they think that religious organizations focus too much on rules and not enough on spirituality, or that religious leaders are too focused on money and power rather than truth and spirituality."[39] Interestingly, very "few say they became unaffiliated because they believe that modern science proves that religion is just superstition."[40] What this research shows is that more people are questioning their religions, but that doesn't necessarily send them to atheism. Instead, it usually sends them to other religions. Luis E. Lugo, one of Pew's lead analysts, notes that one of the main difficulties for religion today is dealing with a potential "decrease in brand loyalty."[41]

Clearly, then, the more education and experience an individual gets, the more likely it is that faith will be questioned, leading to greater churn within religious communities. As individuals live longer, they will have more time to see their chosen religion in action and to decide if they are getting spiritual satisfaction. Whereas people might change religions once, twice, or three times during their life now, that number could rise substantially as health spans extend. Reasons to switch religions could include something a religious organization does that the individual rejects (such as the pedophilia problems within the Catholic church), or it could be more personal, such as marrying someone with a different, and stronger, faith. Such dynamics will no doubt intensify competition among religions for believers, potentially creating even more tension than already exists among the various faiths, including atheism. In other words, longer lives will carry with them a higher risk of religious tension.

THE APPEAL OF RELIGION

Understanding the allure of religion is a complex task. Sigmund Freud and others focused on death anxiety, but that is not the full story. Religion also answers questions about the meaning of life, and, as Aristotle put it, "all men by nature desire to know." We could even argue that as people live longer, they will become more interested in the "meaning of it all." Chapter 6 demonstrated that humans who live longer, healthier lives will also be wealthier. This wealth could allow those who are motivated to "discover the meaning of life" to actually take time to more carefully investigate because they won't be struggling to feed themselves or put a roof over their heads. This scenario is in line with Abraham Maslow's theory that more "actualized" people (basic needs are met) are more likely to have "peak" or mystical experiences.[42] Even Norris and Inglehart note that, while traditional religious practices may erode in wealthier countries, the drive to find the meaning and purpose of life does not.[43]

To the extent that religions can maintain their image as the "go-to" place to find the meaning of life and truth, they will likely have a strong future. Yet even if leaders in the current religious marketplace don't provide what people are looking for, religion will likely still survive in some form because a strong case can be made that no matter what happens, humans are biologically "wired for God." A somewhat humorous example of this tendency was recounted by New York Times columnist Nicholas D. Kristof: "It's striking how faith is almost irrepressible. While I was living in China in the early 1990's, after religion had been suppressed for decades, drivers suddenly began dangling pictures of Chairman Mao from their rear-view mirrors. The word had spread that Mao's spirit could protect them from car crashes or even bring them sons and wealth. It was a miracle: ordinary Chinese had transformed the great atheist into a god."[44] How it is that humans manage to integrate religion into their lives, even in the most unlikely situations?

Harvard biologist and Pulitzer Prize winner Edward O. Wilson first proposed a biological basis for religion in the 1970s and has extended that theory to a range of human cultural practices.[45] Being religious causes individuals to favor group interests over their own, which is thought to have enhanced human survival. "Ethical and religious beliefs are created from the bottom up, from people to their culture," Wilson argues. "They do not come from the top down, from God or other nonmaterial source to the people by way of culture."[46] This idea—that religion has a genetic basis—has spurred research into how our biology is wired for belief. For instance, in 2004 geneticist Dean Hamer wrote a controversial book called *The God Gene* in which he argued that the gene VMAT2 relates to self-transcendence.[47] People with this gene, he proposed, tend to be more spiritual. Other scientists have focused on particular regions of the brain, looking for "God Spots" or "God Modules." Parts of the brain that seem to have some impact on religious experience include the parietal lobe, the prefrontal cortex, and the temporal lobe.[48]

THE CHANGING RELIGIOUS LANDSCAPE

While people will continue to be religious once the threat of death and the promise of the afterlife are no longer "top-of-the-mind" issues, this paradigm shift will no doubt lead to changes in the religious landscape. To use the economic metaphor again, emphasizing the afterlife to gain consumers will no longer be a fruitful approach for religious providers. The question then becomes, how will this affect the religious marketplace? Will religions be forced to evolve? Will new ones crop up? The answer to these questions appears to be yes.

In reality, religion has always been evolving. This might come as a surprise to those who grew up in a religious tradition that emphasized the truth of sacred books and also to atheists who have trouble understanding how someone could remain religious when their main religious text says that it is ok to stone your children to death if they disobey you. For instance, Deuteronomy 21:18–21 asserts:

> If a man have a stubborn and rebellious son, which will not obey the voice of his father, or the voice of his mother, and that, when they have chastened him, will not hearken unto them: Then shall his father and his mother lay hold on him, and bring him out unto the elders of his city, and unto the gate of his place; And they shall say unto the elders of his city, This our son is stubborn and rebellious, he will not obey our voice; he is a glutton, and a drunkard. And all the men of his city shall stone him with stones, that he die: so shalt thou put evil away from among you; and all Israel shall hear, and fear.

Of course, most Christians wouldn't endorse killing their disobedient children or completing any number of other violent actions that are outlined in the Bible but today are seen as barbaric. Instead, most will argue that times have changed and that although the Bible is an important text, not everything in it can be taken literally—some stories are more mythical or literary in nature. Author Dinesh D'Souza explains the apparent quandary this way: "we routinely speak of scientific progress. . . . Religion too can progress. No one is saying that truth itself changes—remember that the principle of relativity operated for billions of years before Einstein discovered it—but our human understanding of truth can and does."[49] The notion that our understanding of truth evolves over time enables religious leaders to reinterpret sacred texts without appearing to be simply following popular opinion. Bishop William E. Swing, a leading force in ordaining both women and gays in the Episcopal church, provides a relatively recent example of truth discovery.

"I ordained more women and more openly gay people than any other bishop in the history of the world-wide church," he said in an interview.[50] As the bishop of the Diocese of California from 1980 to 2006 and based in San Francisco at Grace Cathedral, he had ample opportunity to get to know individuals within the city's very large gay community. He is proud of his work and explains that, even though official Catholic dogma states that "gays are intrinsically disordered," he argues instead that "gays are human beings" who can and do become loyal members of the Christian faith. His work at finding new truths has not stopped there. Bishop Swing has gone on to found the influential United Religions Initiative (URI), an international nongovernmental organization with projects in over seventy countries. URI's mission is to promote interfaith cooperation because, as Swing points out, there "will never be peace among nations unless there is peace among religions."

Bishop Swing is a leader who inspires positive action and mutual respect. He understands that faith can and does evolve, and his advice to others is this: "the trick of leadership is to allow humans to be humans. . . . All religions will have to elevate their game to thrive in the universes that are out there."[51] That is good advice, and a number of religious scholars have begun thinking about how, in a world of longer-lived humans, religion might evolve to fit our enhanced understanding of truth.

STAYING RELEVANT

As we have already discovered, the Christian religion has evolved substantially, but it is not alone. All religions change over time. For instance, in the Jain religion monks and nuns typically "renounce" the world to purify their karma. There are many rules that renouncers adhere to, and for a long time none of them traveled by vehicle because it would have broken the vow of nonviolence (vehicles kill insects and other small forms of life).[52] Renouncers therefore walked everywhere, but this left the international Jain community with limited access to these important individuals. To fix this problem, Sherry Fohr explains, the Jains created a new institution of lesser renouncers who were allowed to travel by vehicles. This was a step toward modernizing Jainism, and Fohr attempts to predict how Jainism might incorporate radical longevity into its mind-set. She posits that Jains could interpret "the longer life spans of humans, resulting from radical life extension technology, as the result of humans' better *ayus* (life) karma that was fixed in their previous lives."[53] And for those unable to afford access to life-extension technologies, it would be thought by many that karma from their last life wasn't good enough and that they needed to build it up now. She also explains that the Jains believe that "no one is innocent; everyone receives what they deserve based on their past actions."[54]

When it comes to the Jewish religion, Rabbi Dorff provides some specific ideas for how Jewish life might morph to fit the realities of a longer-lived membership. "One could imagine synagogues with programs for those from, say, 100–120, 120–140, and so on."[55] Of course, he notes that this assumes "the current desire of people to associate with people of their own generation" once health spans are extended.[56] Writing on behalf of the reformed Protestant perspective, Nigel M. de S. Cameron and Amy Michelle DeBaets predict even more substantial modifications. "There might be movements within the church to change the nature of marriage to something less permanent, as serial episodes in parallel with new career patterns."[57] Such a move would certainly be a theological departure from the current "until death do us part" idea, but it is certainly a possibility once the duration of life expectancies is longer.

There is also potential for Islam to evolve its theology with the advent of life-extension technologies, says Florida International University professor Aisha Y. Musa. Already, a movement is afoot by some Islamic thinkers to view heaven (Jannah) and hell (Jahannam) not as localities but as states of mind. According to theorists such as Ghulam

Ahmed Parvez, heaven "stands for fruition coupled with a glowing home for the future. Hell is the experience of frustration tinged with remorse and regret."[58] Such a reinterpretation of heaven and hell would make radical life-extension work well with Muslim doctrines, Musa argues, and a longer life would certainly offer "Muslims more opportunities to attain knowledge, gain wisdom, and practice piety."[59]

Extending health spans not only will mean more time to examine age-old questions such as the meaning of life but will also present opportunities to start asking *new* questions. Among these, predicts Daoist expert and Boston University religious studies professor Livia Kohn, will be "what is to be done with all that free time and how should one structure a life on earth that has already achieved what used to be the ultimate goal [virtual immortality]?"[60] She goes on to predict that demand for spiritual guidance will be strong because coming to terms with social changes will cause people to "look to philosophers for a new way of thinking that emphasizes cooperation, calmness, and going with the flow."[61] There will also be room to create new rituals for major life transitions such as "from the fourth divorce to the fifth marriage or from their third advanced degree to their next career."[62] Kohn clearly sees life extension as a great opportunity for Daoists to gain a larger share of the religious market because they have always argued that "death and aging are essentially avoidable, and that life in a perfect and harmonious society, where one is paid for realizing oneself and having fun, is the way to go."[63]

That a particular religion already fits well with reality does not guarantee success in obtaining followers. Using rational choice theory, Lawrence Iannaccone explains how strict religious orders, which ask their members to dress in strange ways or follow rules that limit chances for social and economic advancement, remain able to attract members. It seems counterintuitive that such burdens would make a church stronger, but Iannaccone explains it this way: "strictness makes organizations stronger and more attractive because it reduces free riding. It screens out members who lack commitment and stimulates participation among those who remain."[64] In essence, the devout person is willing to pay a high social price because it buys a better religious product. Those who do commit to the religion tend to be passionate, deeply involved in each other's lives, willing to come to each other's aid, are reverential of the same texts, and share common dreams.

Because religion is social by nature, Iannaccone explains, "it is a 'commodity' that people produce collectively."[65] That means that the entire experience relies not just on the individual but also on the inputs of others. Weeding out people who are not committed to the cause enhances the experience. This helps explain why fundamentalist churches in America still thrive even though they reject the scientifically validated reality of evolution. Of course, strictness can go too far, and at some point the disadvantages of zealotry outweigh the benefits, such as when a church doesn't offer substitutes for the items that members are expected to do without. This brings up the question, then, of the essential elements that make something a religion. It's a complicated subject to be sure, but some reasonable answers are possible, and these lead to interesting ideas for future spiritual movements that might compete with the traditional ones we are all familiar with today.

BROADENING RELIGION
IN A LONGER-LIVED WORLD

Religious people are spiritual, but are spiritual people necessarily religious? It's a tough question. According to psychologists Ralph Hood, Peter Hill, and Bernard Spilka, spirituality can be seen as "more personal and psychological than institutional." So when someone says she is "spiritual but not religious," she might mean that she believes in God but rejects traditional religious institutions. Religiousness is also more social. According to Emory University religious history professor Gary Laderman, "Religion is a ubiquitous feature of cultural life" and is "not necessarily about God."[66] What it is always about, however, is the "sacred," which is, as Laderman puts it, a word signifying "communities tied together emotionally and cognitively, but also spiritually and materially by vital rituals, living myths, indescribable experiences, moral values, shared memories, and other commonly recognized features of religious life."[67] Hood, Hill, and Spilka's extensive psychological data agree with this outlook; they note that there are three key aspects to understanding the role of religion in human life. These are the cognitive, the motivational, and the social. With these baseline items, it is possible to discover religious movements outside the traditional venues.

What would constitute examples of unexpected religious movements? Laderman provides an extensive list. He writes that there are religious practices and commitments in "science and the pursuit of truth, music and the social effervescence at concerts, violence and glorification of warfare, celebrity worship and technological wonders; heroic doctors and evil villains, funeral spectacles and sexual compulsions; the Superbowl and sacrificed soldiers; Elvis and drugs, both legal and illegal."[68] An interesting example is Oprah Winfrey as "a source of religious mythology in celebrity culture" who is "at the center of a range of devotional practices that demonstrate the depth and breadth of her religious standing in this prominent culture of worship."[69] Indeed, the rituals that Oprah religionists engage in include watching her talk show; reading her magazine, Web site, and titles from her book club; donating money and time through her Angel Network; and, perhaps most importantly, "journaling at her suggestion for greater self-awareness."[70] Such is the power of this movement that not only is Oprah a very rich woman, but she also inadvertently elicits defensiveness from those involved in traditional religious enterprises. For instance, a YouTube video titled "The Church of Oprah Exposed" accuses Oprah of establishing a cult and LivePrayer.com's Bill Keller has intoned that Oprah's views are like "spiritual crack."[71] These are harsh words for someone who many people see as simply a successful talk show host. But Laderman explains how Oprah's hardcore fans' seemingly regular activities really do have religious dimensions that clearly threaten the religious right.

According to Laderman, "Rituals are religious when they establish order for participants who return to them again and again, bind groups of disparate people into a unified community fixed on a common symbol or totem, empower individuals through expectations of personal transformation, transcendence, and fulfillment including but not limited to physical, embodied experiences, and teach followers about what is really real, especially meaningful, and genuinely insightful."[72] Of course, Oprah is not the only example of new religious movements taking hold where we might least expect them.

Another source of religious fervor is a movement called "transhumanism" (also known as Humanity plus or H+), whose members expect to use technology to transcend the biological limitations of humankind, including death. Not all people who think transhumanism is a good idea can be considered religious. It is possible to support the use of technology to increase human health spans and decrease human suffering without making such ideas life's centerpiece.[73] What makes someone religious is determined by how he allows specific ideas and movements to affect his actions, social groups, and daily rituals. That said, East Carolina University religious studies professor Calvin Mercer, a leading figure in exploring religion and transhumanism, notes that even though "many transhumanists bristle at the thought that their notions have anything to do with religion, . . . I think implicit religious themes can and often are there and when present are certainly worthy of inquiry."[74] We will now examine how religious themes exist within a pro-science movement called the Singularity, a subset of transhumanism.

Ray Kurzweil, a brilliant inventor and futurist, has authored a number of books that could be taken together as religious texts in a "religion of transhumanism." One of his more famous books, *The Singularity Is Near*, discusses the religious nature of his scientific ideas more precisely than one might expect. The book includes an interesting dialog with Microsoft cofounder Bill Gates in which Kurzweil argues, "We need a new religion."[75] When Gates asks what a new religion might look like, Kurzweil provides a detailed answer that his entire book is built around, embodying two principles: "the respect for human consciousness" and "the importance of knowledge."[76] Kurzweil makes it clear that information itself is not knowledge. Instead, knowledge is "information that has meaning for conscious entities: music, art, literature, science, technology." Even though Kurzweil maintains that "singularitianism is not a system of beliefs or unified viewpoints" and that the "last thing we need is another dogma" or cult, a close reading of his work reveals all the elements of a new religion.[77]

The singularity, according to Kurzweil, is "a future period during which the pace of technological change will be so rapid, its impact so deep, that human life will be irreversibly transformed."[78] In effect, he predicts the transcendence of humanity—an element of all traditional religions. But he really builds the foundation for a religious movement by discussing his personal philosophy, which fills in the rest of the blanks for anyone interested in joining. The book even starts with a discussion of his religious upbringing and the first time he imagined that a computer could think. Aside from the title of "singularitarian," he calls himself a "patternist" who "views patterns of information as the *fundamental reality*" (my italics).[79] He argues that he knows the purpose of the universe, which "reflects the same purpose as our lives: to move toward greater intelligence and knowledge."[80] He also tells Bill Gates that "God" is on the way: "Once we saturate the matter and energy in the universe with intelligence," he says "it will 'wake up,' be conscious, and sublimely intelligent. That's about as close to God as I can imagine."[81]

For those wondering what rituals this religion might have, aside from reading the relevant texts and attending singularitarian and trans-humanist-themed conferences, big ones include carefully taking vitamin supplements, exercising, and perhaps even signing up for cryonics and wearing a bracelet identifying oneself as a member of a group whose body or head will be preserved at death in order to be brought back to life when technology makes it possible. Kurzweil even coauthored a book called *Transcend* that offers readers a detailed plan for how to "live long enough to live forever."[82] There is a clear vision of good and evil in this world. Goodness is found in knowledge; evil is death because it is the termination of pattern, a form of knowledge. Although this religion is clearly based on science, faith still comes into play. Kurzweil explains, "I don't know for sure that anything exists other than my own thoughts," and it's "my personal leap of faith" that "I believe in the existence of the universe."[83]

The argument that singularitarianism can be viewed as religion doesn't mean that it is wrong or somehow less legitimate. In a YouTube video taken at a conference where Kurzweil was speaking, a bright-eyed John Heylin attempts to get him to say whether or not his ideas constitute a religion. Kurzweil doesn't answer directly but coyly suggests that "the singularity should not be lumped in with 'pre-scientific or un-scientific' religion."[84] Clearly misunderstanding his comments, the person who posted the YouTube video gave it the title "Ray Kurzweil: The Singularity Is Not a Religion." Although it might indeed be true that "being a singularitarian is not a matter of faith" and that Kurzweil did not come to his "perspective as a result of searching for an alternative to customary faith," it is true that all the elements of a postscientific religious movement exist in spades.[85] As Kurzweil writes, "We can regard, therefore, the freeing of our thinking from the severe limitations of its biological form to be an essential spiritual undertaking."[86]

This exercise of looking at how singularitarians or transhumanists have built a set of ideas that can be modeled into a working religion demonstrates what at least one strong contemporary religion looks like, and it provides clues to the older religions about how they can focus to compete. The essential elements outlined here include a vision of good and evil, promises of transcendence, prescribed rituals, and answers to the purpose of life and the universe. Not only can religion exist in a postscientific world, then, but it also can be modeled quite nicely on science itself.

Humans appear to be wired for religion, so it is unlikely to fade, but it will change forms as health spans extend and death becomes less of a factor in the human paradigm. New religions will form, and older religions will be wise to carefully examine their congregations' needs if they wish to survive in the religious marketplace. In the end, we can say that even if the secularists are wrong that religion will fade, so are traditional religious leaders if they believe that the afterlife will continue to be the force it has historically been. Who, then, is leading the charge into this new paradigm, and should it be embraced? That is the subject of the next chapter.

CHAPTER 8

Leadership for a
Longer-Lived World

T HIS BOOK BEGAN with a discussion of humanity's enduring desire
for longer and healthier lives—a powerful dream that is deeply
ingrained in our culture. Dreams are the seeds of change, but for those
seeds to grow into reality, directed action is necessary. In this chapter
we will examine some of the leaders whose efforts have brought us to
where we are now. We will also look at why there is still more to be
done. In Chapter 2 we discovered brilliant scientists whose breakthroughs will improve health and revolutionize medicine. But change
is not driven by science alone. For longevity science to be funded,
accepted, and embraced, a cultural shift also has to happen. Achieving the dream, then, requires a diverse ecosystem of people and institutions working together to affect societal "memes," or ways of
thinking. This enterprise has already begun.

"All over the world and right in your backyard, there are people
who are steadily pushing back the frontier of aging. They are not
content to simply wither away, becoming frail and feeling worthless,"
says CNN's Dr. Sanjay Gupta.[1] Dr. Gupta is one of the people leading the charge in spreading the meme that healthy life extension is
not only a possibility but is also worth fighting for. A neurosurgeon
and chief medical correspondent for CNN, he is on the front lines

when it comes to discovering and explaining cutting-edge science. Former president Bill Clinton calls him "the world's doctor," and the public relies on him to separate medical fact from fiction. Aside from his regular news reports, Dr. Gupta has written a couple of books that explain how advances in science are promoting health extension. His message is that there is a tsunami of longevity-related research in the works and that "there is nothing more important."[2] Dr. Gupta might think of himself as simply a doctor who is informing the public about new advances, but when it comes to explaining how the longevity meme has caught on, we could call him a "salesperson."

Labeling Dr. Gupta a salesperson is not derogatory. He is obviously not trying to "sell" a product in return for money. Rather, the term is derived from Malcolm Gladwell's best-selling book *The Tipping Point*, in which he explains how certain people and circumstances come together to make an idea unstoppable. In this context a salesperson is someone who exudes energy, enthusiasm, and charm, someone who can effectively and charismatically explain concepts and ideas.[3] Of course, Dr. Gupta isn't alone in this role. Society has reached a longevity tipping point because many players are involved.

SALESPEOPLE:
SPREADING THE MEME

"Here's our plan for living to 125!" announced Oprah Winfrey when interviewing eighty-five-year-old billionaire businessman David Murdock.[4] Her show examined the benefits of caloric restriction, and although Murdock didn't actually count calories, the way he ate ensured that he consumed significantly less than the average American. Oprah's shows on longevity together with her endorsement of doctors like Mehmet Oz have done much to educate the public and popularize the idea of healthy life extension.

Dr. Oz, a cardiothoracic surgeon and host of the popular *Dr. Oz Show*, is a solid leader and salesperson for the longevity meme. He is charming and charismatic, and his books, shows, and Web sites about how to live better explicitly promote health extension. Not only that, but he and his frequent coauthor, Dr. Michael Roizen, take the idea of antiaging a step further with the Web site RealAge.com. One of the goals of RealAge.com is to highlight the difference between *chronological* age and *biological* age: the number of years someone is alive verses how fast she has aged. The message is that life choices affect how fast a body deteriorates and that there are actions that can be taken to slow down the damage so as to extend health span. This focus is refreshing because typically the media tend to concentrate mostly on cosmetic issues.

One of the most radical means to achieve greater longevity is caloric restriction, or limiting calories while increasing nutrients. As we learned in Chapter 2, this type of diet has been shown to cause changes that significantly slow down aging. In discussing the topic, Dr. Oz told Oprah's audience that it is possible to talk about "very specifically allowing us to go into our second century of life with the vitality and the bounciness that you have when you're a young person."[5] In fact, he said that Joe Cordell, a man who practices caloric restriction and who Dr. Oz interviewed in the audience that day, "may become the first man in history to live to be 150 years old."[6] That is an exciting message, and Dr. Oz is leading the way in showing the public that the science has now advanced to a point where these kinds of claims have legitimacy. And his coverage of the topic doesn't end there. In conjunction with Oprah, he has discussed regenerative medicine and the fact that scientists can now rebuild body parts in order to maintain health. On this issue Dr. Oz said, "These are technologies that fascinate me because they could add decades to our life."[7] Oprah marveled at the advances, and in looking at the reality that researchers have already "grown nearly two dozen different types of body parts, including muscle, bones and a working heart valve," the talk show host enthusiastically remarked that "you used to read about this in science fiction and couldn't even imagining it happening."[8] Indeed, things have changed, and charismatic salespeople who deal in ideas are letting the world know.

MAVENS: DATA COLLECTORS
FUELING THE LONGEVITY MEME

While salespeople work to popularize a new meme, those who help build it can be called "mavens." These are the people who are committed to collecting and disbursing information. They are like databanks, almost compulsively collecting and offering data to others who show interest.[9] In the longevity movement, there are a lot of these types of people, ranging from those who are seen as either cutting edge or "fringe" to those who are more mainstream.

One well-known maven is Aubrey de Grey, whom we learned a bit about in Chapter 2. A computer scientist turned gerontologist, de Grey describes himself as a "fighter at heart." He battles aging, he says, because of the suffering it causes. "Aging is just like smoking: It's really bad for you. It shortens your life, it typically makes the last several years of your life rather grim, and it also makes those years pretty hard for your loved ones."[10]

After becoming interested in aging theory, de Grey spent three years doing extensive research, culminating in a book titled *The Mitochondrial Free Radical Theory of Aging*, which impressed folks at Cambridge University so much that they awarded him a PhD.[11] But that was only the beginning of this maven's quest. After deciding that aging didn't necessarily need to be understood but that it just needed to be *fixed*, he came up with his SENS theory, described in Chapter 2. Since architecting the SENS strategy, de Grey has done everything he can to spread the word and says that on average he does two media interviews a week.[12] He has appeared on television shows such as *60 Minutes*, CNN's *Vital Signs* with Dr. Sanjay Gupta, and even *The Colbert Report*. He gave a talk at the prestigious TED (Technology, Entertainment, and Design) conference, and he organizes his own conferences to bring together scientists in the field to discuss breakthroughs and brainstorm over how to implement the SENS blueprint. He is a man obsessed with collecting and sharing data on how to repair human beings. GQ magazine described him this way: "he analyzes other people's work, charts the innovations and disappointments from hundreds of labs across dozens of disciplines. Then he synthesizes all this information and applies what's pertinent to his grand idea."[13] This is typical maven activity, and without it, the field would have trouble moving forward. Indeed, recognizing the value of collecting and synthesizing data has led some thinkers to argue that more advanced computers are needed to more quickly learn how to repair the damage of aging.

Dr. Ben Goertzel, CEO of two artificial intelligence (AI) companies and supervisor at a robotics lab at Xiamen University in China, is a maven who spends a good deal of brainpower thinking about the intersection of artificial intelligence and aging. In his paper "AI Against Aging," Dr. Goertzel explains how his team used AI to "discover the genetic basis of Chronic Fatigue Syndrome, and to create novel diagnostics for Parkinson's disease based on identifying subtle patterns of damage in mitochondrial DNA."[14] The human body, while complex, is ultimately a machine, Goertzel argues. This means it is both modifiable and reparable, but the biggest problem Goertzel sees is that we have too much data and not enough human bandwidth to analyze everything. "The human brain simply was not evolved for the integrative analysis of a massive number of complexly-interrelated, high-dimensional biological datasets," he writes.[15] "In the short term, the most feasible path to working around this problem is to supplement human biological scientists with increasingly advanced AI software, gradually moving toward the goal of an AGI (Artificial General Intelligence) bioscientist."[16] Just as Google is a form of artificial intelligence that allows for fast searching of the Internet, a software program that could "read" biological studies and help to sort the data for human scientists would make the task of finding repair mechanisms for the human body that much easier.

Another proponent of this idea is maven Ray Kurzweil. In 1999 President Bill Clinton awarded Ray Kurzweil the National Medal of Technology, the highest honor for technological achievement bestowed by the president of the United States on America's leading innovators. Microsoft cofounder Bill Gates has called Kurzweil "the best person I know at predicting the future of artificial intelligence." Incredibly prolific, Kurzweil was the principal developer of the first print-to-speech reading machine for the blind, the first CCD flat-bed scanner, the first text-to-speech synthesizer, the first music synthesizer capable of re-creating the grand piano and other orchestral instruments, and the first commercially marketed, large-vocabulary speech recognition technology.[17] That is, it's safe to say that he is good at collecting information and translating it into usable ideas and products.

In his book *The Singularity Is Near*, Kurzweil discusses how exponentially growing technology will have many important effects, such as pushing the growth of AI that will help humans solve longevity problems. He writes, "Human life expectancy is itself growing steadily and will accelerate rapidly, now that we are in the early stages of reverse engineering the information processes underlying life and disease. Robert Freitas estimates that eliminating a specific list comprising 50 percent of medically preventable conditions would extend human life expectancy to over 150 years."[18] It is this authoritative tone and well-researched work that makes Kurzweil and his 650-page book a big hit with those looking for detailed and dependable information. This work was published on the heels of another book that he had coauthored with fellow maven and longevity expert Dr. Terry Grossman. In *Fantastic Voyage: Live Long Enough to Live Forever*, the pair offer practical advice on how to keep the body healthy using today's limited technology so that a person can live long enough to take advantage of regenerative medicine and other scientific advances in the future.[19] Indeed, Kurzweil's work as a maven is so respected that a new university, based at NASA's Moffett Field in California, was named Singularity University, and he was appointed chancellor. (People often confuse Singularity University with the philosophical movement "singularitarianism," but the two are not the same, as indicated in Chapter 7.)

SU's mission is practical: "to assemble, educate and inspire leaders who strive to understand and facilitate the development of exponentially advancing technologies in order to address humanity's grand challenges."[20] The academic tracks are geared toward understanding how fast-moving technologies can work together, and more than half of them have a direct impact on the field of longevity research. These tracks include AI and robotics; nanotechnology, networks, and computing systems; biotechnology and bioinformatics; medicine and neuroscience; and futures studies and forecasting.[21] SU is a place where mavens speak to those who are superfocused on changing the world for the better. It is no surprise, then, that it also functions as an institutional "connector"—the third component needed to successfully spread a game-changing meme.

CONNECT ME

Peter Diamandis always seems to be on the phone or leaving a meeting to get on a phone call. His calendar is littered with birthday reminders on practically every day.[22] He is the chairman and cofounder of Singularity University, and he is what many would call a "connector"— someone who knows lots of people.[23] Always full of energy, Diamandis clearly enjoys networking and relentlessly connects with different types of people day in and day out. This skill is the third part of the leadership team that brings about significant social change. When it comes to the longevity meme, at least two of Diamandis's nonprofit start-ups are making a direct impact.

In addition to SU, Diamandis's other relevant nonprofit for longevity science is the X PRIZE, which was originally focused on space. The X PRIZE, an incentive prize, began by offering $10 million for "the first privately financed team that could build a three-passenger vehicle and fly it 100 kilometers into space twice within a 2-week period."[24] Since that prize was successfully won by Burt Rutan (backed by Microsoft cofounder Paul Allen), the organization has branched out to tackle other issues. The second prize is a $10 million Archon Genomics X PRIZE. Why genomics? As Diamandis puts it, "Our goal is to greatly reduce the cost, and increase the speed of, human genome sequencing. This achievement will unleash a new era of personalized, predictive and preventive medicine, eventually transforming medical care from reactive to proactive."[25] In an interview on the subject, Diamandis says, "Personally, I am excited to be alive during a period of human evolution where we have the potential to extend life indefinitely."[26]

A physician by training, Diamandis's interest in longevity was sparked, he says, in his twenties when he watched a television program about turtles, according to which some species can lives hundreds of years. "I thought, if they can live that long, why can't I?"[27] These are the type of big questions he likes to ask, and he usually does it in the company of big names. When he was interviewed for this book, he had just returned from a "Zero-G" flight with Hollywood director James Cameron and had recently met with X PRIZE Genomics cochair Dr. J. Craig Venter, of Human Genome Project fame.

Whether he thinks about it or not, Diamandis is clearly leveraging his relationships to promote the healthy longevity meme. Supporters of the Genomics X PRIZE listed on the organization's Web site include theoretical physicist Professor Stephen Hawking and former CNN interview show host Larry King. Connected to the cause by Diamandis, both Hawking and King act as salespeople for the cause.[28] For instance, Hawking says, "You may know that I am suffering from what is known as Amyotrophic Lateral Sclerosis (ALS), or Lou Gehrig's Disease, which is thought to have a genetic component to its origin. It is for this reason that I am a supporter of the $10M Archon Genomics X PRIZE to drive rapid human genome sequencing. This prize and the resulting technology can help bring about an era of personalized medicine."[29] Larry King goes straight to the point when he asks, "What if we could learn how to stop heart disease from happening? What if we were able to reduce a person's likelihood of cardiovascular disease based on his or her genetic profile, as well as on the individual's age, gender, and lifestyle?"[30] King continues, "It is my hope that by supporting the Archon Genomics X PRIZE to drive rapid human genome sequencing that we can get answers to these questions and help our Foundation save more lives in the years to come."[31] The message is that healthy life extension is possible, and the Genomics X PRIZE is contributing to achieving that goal.

Just as maven Ray Kurzweil is teamed up with connector Peter Diamandis, until recently Aubrey de Grey was teamed up with entrepreneur David Gobel. After meeting de Grey online in 2000, Gobel was inspired to start a nonprofit to support life-extension efforts, and in 2003 the pair launched the Mprize, which is awarded to either of two categories: "the research team that breaks the world record for the oldest-ever mouse" (longevity) and the research team that creates "the best-ever late-onset intervention" (rejuvenation).[32]

Like Diamandis, Gobel is a big believer in incentive prizes and even goes as far as to say, "If you want to end cancer, what you would need is a 20 billion dollar prize issued by the government. Then it would happen."[33] When questioned about such a large amount, he explains that the innovation coming from the prize (which would not be paid until someone won) would be offset by the savings in Medicare for those dying from the disease. Indeed, considering that the National Cancer Institute reports that "cancer care accounted for an estimated $104.1 billion in medical care expenditures in the United States in 2006," it doesn't seem like such an unreasonable idea.[34]

As for the Mprize, it currently has $3.8 million in its pot, but the prizes do not cash out the entire amount when won, and the prize continues to collect money through donations. Although much smaller than the X PRIZE or potential government-backed prizes, the Mprize has already played an important function in getting researchers to feel comfortable talking about fighting aging. Gobel explains that "the existence of the Mprize and the fact that Aubrey didn't back off [after the MIT challenge] definitely led to a positive sea change in the attitude of longevity and biogerontology researchers who previously may have secretly wanted to push the boundaries faster and harder, but could not and did not do it out of fear of reprisal or cutting off of funding. We noted a real change in the direction away from 'it's preposterous and life extension will never happen' to 'it's going to happen—someday.'"[35] This certainly marks a big milestone on the road leading to acceptance of the longevity meme.

In comparing himself with de Grey, Gobel jokes that he is "a second banana," but in reality they have different skill sets and roles. Although still friendly, the two parted ways in March 2009 seemingly because de Grey is focused on maven-like activities, like funding detailed scientific research, while Gobel is interested in connector-type activities, such as funding shorter-term entrepreneurial ventures like Organovo, a regenerative medicine company that applies proprietary technology to print new organs.[36] Gobel explains the rationale for the organ-printing company in terms of not only how it can make the world a healthier place, but also how it can harness the imagination of an entirely new group of people in favor of health extension. "There are about 2–3 million people in the western world who need new organs and who show up nowhere on any [waiting] lists," he says. "This is the group we are working to engage, and their latent/unharnessed energy is probably 100 times greater than the life-extension community at present."[37] Spoken like a true connector. It is worth noting that connectors are not always attached to one maven; in fact, they usually aren't because they tend to know many mavens.

Christine Peterson is another connector spreading the longevity meme. She cofounded the Foresight Institute for Nanotechnology, which works to promote the upsides, and help avoid the dangers, of nanotechnology and similar life-changing developments.[38] Nanotechnology will play a big role in life-extension efforts in multiple ways, including drug development and biosensors. And even though Peterson is still the president of the Foresight Institute, she also organizes many successful conferences, including one called the Personalized Life Extension Conference: Anti-Aging Strategies for a Long Healthy Life.[39] If that sounds like a fringe conference, think again. The headliner for the event was venture capitalist (VC) Ester Dyson, who sits on the board of directors for genomics company 23andMe and is a former chairman of the illustrious Internet Corporation for Assigned Names and Numbers, the agency governing the Internet address system. Hedge fund manager, VC, and PayPal cofounder Peter Thiel also delivered a keynote, as did multi-prize-winning scientist Bruce Ames, after whom the Ames test for carcinogens is named.

Venture capitalists are now paying close attention to the longevity space. Ester Dyson discussed her interest in an interview with the *New York Times*. "I'm looking at a lot of companies that are in the formation mode of health and self tracking platforms," she said in February 2010.[40] This helps explain why she was speaking at a life-extension conference organized by Peterson, who is superconnected to individuals in that industry. And Dyson isn't alone. At the 2010 Fortune Tech Brainstorm conference in Aspen, investors paid close attention to a panel discussion on "smart biology: where computer science meets health care."[41] Similarly, at the 2010 Techonomy conference in Tahoe, venture capitalists and angel investors discussed what they called the "new biology," among other tech issues.[42] And while some connectors organize conferences, others work on starting companies.

Bruce Klein is a quiet guy with a big database. Not all connectors are big talkers who are always on the phone. Instead, some are quiet "people collectors." As Malcolm Gladwell describes it, this type of connector is "more an observer, with the dry, knowing manner of someone who likes to remain a little bit on the outside."[43] Klein doesn't make a lot of noise, but he does have a lot of friends, and he is willing to go out of his way to help people in need. He has been known to open his home to health extension colleagues getting settled in Silicon Valley, and he and his wife, Susan, were instrumental in helping Ray Kurzweil and Peter Diamandis pull together Singularity University's first group of core supporters.[44] When Klein explained how he keeps track of the thousands of contacts he has, he said, "I keep a master spreadsheet updated," and out of 5,000 or so people, there are "probably between 300 to 500 true 'friends' that I could call on to help."[45] That's a strong social network, which Klein has leveraged many times over the years. First, he started the unconventional-sounding Immortality Institute, and he then moved closer to the mainstream with organizations like Singularity University, of which he was a founding architect. Now, he has cofounded a company with another connector, James Clement. The two are interested in analyzing supercentenarian genomic data to identify and speed the development of longevity therapies. Called Acron Cell, their company has attracted eminent scientist Dr. George Church of Harvard University, who developed the first direct genomic sequencing method in 1984, as an advisor. Clearly, connectors are also cooperators, and the Internet has made that job much easier than it used to be.

"Bruce was always online," said Kevin Perrott, another connector who is working on a PhD in regenerative medicine at the University of Alberta in Canada.[46] As of the writing of this book, Perrott was in California doing lab work at the Buck Institute, where the longevity meme is bolstered by solid scientific research. "I'm a collaborator," he says. "I know that we can't do big things by ourselves."[47] Perrott is well known in health extension circles for a variety of actions, including a stint as executive director of the Mprize. He founded the Aging Research Network, a Canadian charity that sponsors "research to reverse the diseases of aging," and he joined the board of Aubrey de Grey's new SENS Foundation. He also cofounded the LifeStar Institute, an organization dedicated to "highlighting the economic imperatives for the development of therapies for age-related disease."[48] The LifeStar Institute, while new, is supported by Barbara Logan, who was formerly president and COO of ComputerLand Corporation, at one time the world's largest retailer of personal computers.[49] Perrott clearly is on a mission to help people live longer and healthier lives, and he makes a point of saying that in order to get there, a large community of people needs to be rallied and organized. "There are three ways to create a critical mass," he says, "commercial investment, incentive prizes, and changing academic minds."[50] He seems to be working on all three in tandem, which brings us to the next ingredients for social change: the stickiness factor and the power of context.

IS IT REAL, AND ARE
THE COOL KIDS DOING IT?

A meme becomes sticky only if it is both memorable and moves us to action.[51] On the first count, longevity has no problems. Whether consciously or not, living longer, healthier, and more youthfully is a perennial human desire that seems hardwired in most people's brains. This makes the message of the longevity meme very "sticky" so long as it is based in scientific fact. Few are interested in the topic of antiaging if the message is only the musings of a bunch of quacks. Only a *real* possibility of increased health spans will instigate action. Fortunately, as we know, the science has moved forward enough that the idea of living much longer and healthier lives is a real possibility that is starting to get coverage by established media outlets. For instance, Oprah fans were treated to an insider's view of one area of regenerative medicine when Dr. Oz brought an organ mold on the show and demonstrated how it could be lined with cells to create a new body part for one that has broken down. That's a "wow" factor that sticks in people's minds like superglue. This stickiness is part of the larger context, which is also key to spreading a meme.

Ideas that are unstoppable can also be called "social epidemics," and they are "sensitive to the conditions and circumstances of the times and places in which they occur."[52] Gladwell explains this phenomenon in the retail world through the example of Hush Puppy shoes, which, he argues, became popular "because they were being worn by kids in the cutting-edge precincts of the East Village—an environment that helped others to look at the shoes in a new light."[53] So what is the history and who are the 'cool kids' driving the longevity meme?

Arguably, the event that really brought longevity science to the forefront of the public's mind was the dual announcement of the first "completion" of a draft of the human genome in 2000 by both Celera Genomics, a private company founded by Dr. J. Craig Venter, and the Human Genome Project, an international public consortium

backed with around $3 billion U.S. tax dollars.[54] Both President Bill
Clinton and Prime Minister of Britain Tony Blair presided over the
press conference announcing that humanity now possessed "the genetic blueprint for human beings."[55] President Clinton proudly told
the world that the capacity to sequence human genomes "will revolutionize the diagnosis, prevention and treatment of most, if not all,
human diseases."[56] This new ability to look at the "source code" of
humans particularly resonated with computer experts in Silicon Valley and around the world who spend much of their time designing
code for computers. If the source code of humans can be identified,
then it is not that much of a leap to think about re-engineering it.

Suddenly, biology became a field that computer geeks could attempt to tackle, which not only resulted in smart biohackers forming
do-it-yourself biology clubs, but also increased the pace of advances
in biology. Bioinformatics are moving at the speed of Moore's Law
and sometimes faster. To the extent that wealthy technology moguls
influence public opinion and hackers seem cool, the context for the
longevity meme is sizzling hot.

In a *Wired* magazine interview in April 2010, Bill Gates, America's richest man, told reporter Steven Levy that if he were a teenager
today, "he'd be hacking biology."[57] Gates elaborated, saying, "Creating artificial life with DNA synthesis, that's sort of the equivalent of
machine-language programming." Whether or not his comments
were meant as an endorsement of the field, the smart whiz kids
who read *Wired* probably see it that way. And Gates isn't the only
technology mogul to express great interest in biology becoming a
technology project. In a graduation speech at Princeton University,
Amazon.com founder Jeff Bezos told students that "we humans, plod-
ding as we are, will astonish ourselves. . . . Atom by atom we'll assemble small machines that can enter cell walls and make repairs. This
month comes the extraordinary, but inevitable news that we've synthesized life, and in the coming years we'll not only synthesize it, but
engineer it to specifications. I believe you will even see us understand
the human brain. Jules Verne, Mark Twain, Galileo, Newton—all

the curious from the ages would have wanted to be alive most of all right now."[58] That's quite the endorsement of longevity science. Not only is it cool, but also, according to Bezos, top characters from history would have loved to be here to see it. His message, which is true, is that we are living in a time of accelerating change that is going to positively impact the health and longevity of real people alive today.

The synthetic life Bezos was referring to is one of Venter's latest accomplishments. In May 2010 Venter announced that his team had achieved the great feat of creating a synthetic cell. This is "the first self-replicating species we've had on the planet whose parent is a computer," he proclaimed with great fanfare.[59] Because the idea of creating synthetic life pushed some individuals' worry buttons and also annoyed scientists who thought the claim was overstated, Venter spent time afterward explaining exactly what his experiment meant. In a *Wall Street Journal* article, Dr. Venter and molecular biologist Daniel Gibson write, "Even though the cytoplasm of the recipient cell is not synthetic," the bacterium is synthetic "because it is controlled only by a synthetic genome assembled from chemically synthesized pieces of DNA."[60] To explain it in terms computer users might understand, they note that "the DNA software builds its own hardware so that the properties of the cells controlled by the synthetic genome are expected to be the same as if the whole cell had been produced synthetically."[61] This technique could lead to new ways to create vaccines or energy sources. If Bill Gates is right that it would be supercool to have a job creating synthetic life by hacking DNA, then Craig Venter is one of the coolest kids on the block. The context being created here is one in which humans not only dream of manipulating DNA for the betterment of humanity, but also actually do so.

On the "do-it-yourself [DIY] bio" mailing list, composed of self-described "open-source and DIY biology geeks," a hot discussion ensued. "Craig Venter has done it finally!" said one member. "I just wish he had done something cool with it. What he did was use a star trek replicator to bake a cookie," complained another. To which a third member replied, "That's like complaining that Alexander Graham Bell didn't recite Milton into the first phone, instead of saying 'Watson, come here!'"[62] The cool kids in the biohacking world, many of whom have competed at the international genetically engineered machine competition, are not only watching Dr. Venter with great interest; they are also working to create their own projects.

Making cells blink, glow, or smell like banana is what many DIY bio types have on their minds, and such frivolous pursuits are reminiscent of the beginnings of the personal computer revolution. Back in the 1970s, it was the Homebrew Club that brought together clever thinkers—such as future Apple founders Steve Jobs and Steve Wozniak—to trade parts, circuits, and information for DIY computing devices. The point is that biology has become the latest and greatest engineering project, one that hobbyists celebrate. More importantly, eventually this passion will change the world. Those who have already made it big in the technology industry have not failed to notice. Aside from Bill Gates and Jeff Bezos, other tech titans who are driving interest in the longevity meme include Oracle's Larry Ellison, PayPal cofounder Peter Thiel, Google's Larry Page and Sergey Brin, and Microsoft cofounder Paul Allen.

TECH TITANS TAKING ON BIOLOGY

"Death has never made any sense to me," Larry Ellison told investigative reporter Mike Wilson, who wrote an authorized biography of the so-called bad boy of Silicon Valley. "How can a person be there and then just vanish, just not be there? . . . Death makes me very angry. Premature death makes me angrier still."[63] With these sentiments, it's not surprising that Ellison has devoted a large chunk of his wealth to antiaging research. Around 1998 he started the Ellison Foundation, which states on its Web site that its mission is to support "basic biomedical research on aging relevant to understanding life span development processes and age-related diseases and disabilities."[64] Richard Sprott, the foundation's executive director, says that the organization spends around $42 million per year on bioscience donations, and a number of those receiving grants are the hottest names in antiaging work. For instance, the University of California, San Francisco's Dr. Cynthia Kenyon, who discovered life-span-regulating genes, received at least two grants for her work. Likewise, Harvard's Dr. David Sinclair, who started Sirtris Pharmaceuticals to develop a drug based on resveratrol, was awarded at least two grants from the foundation, starting in 2001. As we learned in Chapter 2, in 2008 Sinclair's company was sold to GlaxoSmithKline for $720 million, demonstrating that some of Ellison's antiaging bets are not only edgy but also highly valued by the marketplace. Just as Bill Gates expressed an interest in biology, Ellison also says it could have been an alternate career, going so far as to actually spend two weeks working in the lab of Dr. Joshua Lederberg, the Nobel Prize–winning biologist.[65]

Peter Thiel is another Silicon Valley billionaire who actively supports work on longevity and is propagating the meme of healthy life extension. The PayPal cofounder and venture capitalist was also the first outside investor in Facebook (and was played by actor Wallace Langham in the movie *The Social Network*, starring Jesse Eisenberg and Justin Timberlake). When he's not investing in cool tech companies like Facebook, Thiel is working with his associates at the Founder's Fund to create a unique kind of investment strategy that looks for cutting-edge tech-meets-science projects, such as Halcyon Molecular, which is competing in the gene sequencing space. On the nonprofit side, Thiel has donated significant amounts to Aubrey de Grey's work at the Methuselah Foundation and SENS Foundation as well as to organizations like the Singularity Institute for Artificial Intelligence and Singularity University, among others. When asked about investing in health extension ideas, either for profit or non-profit, Thiel responds, "The great unfinished task of the modern world is to turn death from a fact of life into a problem to be solved—a problem towards whose solution I hope to contribute in whatever way I can."[66]

Larry Page and Sergey Brin of Google are perhaps less direct when it comes to discussing health extension ideas in public, but both are contributing to the meme in various ways. Through Google, Larry Page has given over $250,000 to Singularity University and has said that if he were a student, SU is where he'd want to be.[67] Interestingly, his wife, Lucy Southworth, is a biologist who has written papers on aging issues, including one titled "Effects of Aging on Mouse Transcriptional Networks," coauthored with Stanford's Dr. Stuart K. Kim, who is a well-known aging expert and one of Larry Ellison's award recipients.[68] Sergey Brin is spreading the meme in a more personal way.

23andMe is a genomics company that was cofounded by Brin's biologist wife, Anne Wojcicki, and has gone a long way toward popularizing the idea of personalized medicine. "Spit parties" are one of the cute marketing techniques the company uses to get the public interested in thinking about their DNA and how it might be fixed to cure disease. One high-profile party took place during New York City's Fashion Week. Company staffers recounted the event on their blog, saying, "23andMe managed to lure a few hundred people away from the catwalks Tuesday night to consider the beauty that lies within—DNA. Our Fashion Week spit party was sort of like a Tupperware party, except instead of buying plastic containers the guests were invited to deposit a saliva sample into one. And instead of taking place at a suburban ranch house designed by Richard Neutra, our spit party went down at the spectacular Manhattan headquarters of IAC/InterActive Corporation, designed by architect Frank Gehry."[69] Such hip parties showcasing how biology meets technology are key in spreading the meme of health extension. All the cool kids are doing it.

Of course, sometimes examining DNA leads a person to find out things about his genes that cause concern, and that's where Sergey Brin's biggest public contribution to the meme comes in. It turns out that he has a mutation on one of his genes that makes it 30 to 75 percent more likely that he will develop Parkinson's disease, a neurological condition that interferes with movement, speech, and other functions. His mother already has the disease and has the same mutation.[70] Since learning about his predisposition, Brin has reportedly contributed some $50 million to the cause, which is in addition to the $3.9 million Google invested in 23andMe after Brin made an initial loan of $2.6 million.[71] It is worth pointing out here that Brin is not a wealthy man who has Parkinson's; he's a wealthy man who *might* get Parkinson's. The idea of preemptively funding work into diseases an individual is predisposed to is a sea change from how medical donations traditionally work. But that's not all that's changed.

In a world where biology is technology, the method of gathering data and acting on it may also differ. In a June 2010 interview, Brin told *Wired* magazine's Thomas Goetz, "Generally the pace of medical research is glacial compared to what I'm used to in the Internet. We could be looking lots of places and collecting lots of information. And if we see a pattern, that could lead somewhere."[72] Goetz therefore correctly observed, "Brin is proposing to bypass centuries of scientific epistemology in favor of a more Googley kind of science. He wants to collect data first, then hypothesize, and then find the patterns that lead to answers."[73] Clearly, engineers are getting their hands wet in the biology area, and this has even forced some mavens to rethink how they talk about the subject. Mike Kope, the CEO of Aubrey de Grey's SENS Foundation, says that the organization's message is now quite simple: "repair the damage, don't chase the pathology."[74] And although science has made excellent progress when it comes to understanding body parts like the kidney and heart, the brain remains too complicated to fully comprehend. That's where Microsoft cofounder Paul Allen has decided to contribute.

"Over the last decade I have become increasingly interested in the fields of genomics and neuroscience, and their important role in human development, behavior, and health—and ultimately, understanding more about how the brain actually works," Allen said when he announced his commitment of $100 million in seed money for brain research and the Allen Institute for Brain Science in Seattle.[75] If humans are able to live longer, they are going to need brains that can keep up with the rest of their bodies. For instance, Alzheimer's, a brain disease that affects memory and behavior mainly in older people, is the seventh leading cause of death in the United States and is only set to get worse if new therapies and a cure are not found. In September 2006 the Allen Institute completed a three-dimensional map of gene expression in the mouse brain, which is significant not only because mice share 90 percent of their genes with humans, but also because mapping is the first step toward the goal of reverse engineering. In 2008 the institute announced that it was moving forward with plans to map the human brain, an "atlas that overlays information about gene activity onto a three-dimensional anatomic map."[76] This is exciting, said neurosurgeon Dr. Greg Foltz of the Swedish Medical Center in Seattle, because "the human brain atlas will provide a critical resource for any scientist or physician interested in treating diseases of the brain."[77] The institute is giving away all its information for free to researchers around the world, which should help speed up discoveries in this area. Following this initiative, the National Institutes of Health (NIH) announced in 2009 that it was awarding $30 million to launch the "Human Connectome Project," which will map the circuitry of the healthy adult human brain.[78] This is different from the Allen Institute's work in that it focuses on anatomical details, like the size of synaptic vesicles, instead of genes. And these are not the only projects aimed at understanding the brain. IBM's Dharmendra Modha, whose work has received millions in funding from the Defense Advanced Research Projects Agency, says he is trying to "engineer the mind by reverse engineering the brain," and the "Blue Brain Project" based in Switzerland (using an IBM supercomputer) aims "to reverse-engineer the mammalian brain, in order to understand brain function and dysfunction through detailed simulations."[79]

NECESSITY AS CONTEXT

Clearly, the cool factor of Silicon Valley is helping to spread the longevity meme, but there is another aspect to the context or environment that is helping to spread this meme faster than it would otherwise travel. Although almost cliché to note, this factor is an important part of the equation. That is, there is a large aging population that is wealthy and willing to spend a lot of money on anything that will help it stay healthier longer. Usually, this story is told in the context of spoiled baby-boomers who, used to getting everything they want, now want to defeat death. The reality is more complex than that.

The boomers happen to be alive at a time when technology has developed to a point where it is possible to speak realistically about interventions to prolong health span. It is also the case that the older population is growing faster than the younger population, which creates an urgent economic imperative to find ways to solve the problems of aging so that the health care system doesn't collapse under the weight of a large number of sick people and so that the economy doesn't lose large numbers of workers. As the *New York Times* pointed out in an October 2010 article, "For the first time in human history, people aged 65 and over are about to outnumber children under 5."[80] This "gray tsunami" has worried many policy makers and caused Standard and Poor's to release a report suggesting that without government action, "sovereign debt could become unsustainable, rivaling levels seen during cataclysms like the Great Depression and World War II."[81]

These potentially harsh implications associated with global aging have not been lost on those promoting the longevity meme. In July 2010 a group of longevity scientists, including the eminent (and late) Dr. Robert Butler, released a paper arguing that "to preempt a global aging crisis, we advocate an ambitious global initiative to translate these [longevity science] findings into interventions for aging humans."[82] It is time to change national priorities when it comes to funding disease research, they argue, because although it has always been known that disease risk increases with age, it is now known that "aging is plastic." This means that "within a species, maximum life span is not fixed but can be increased by dietary manipulation [particularly caloric restriction] or genetic manipulation."[83] If researchers could figure out how to translate these lab results into therapies for humans, it would significantly "alleviate the projected social costs and challenge of global demographic aging."[84] Such an argument is similar to the one advanced in 2006 by epidemiologist S. Jay Olshansky, Alliance for Aging Research executive Daniel Perry, and others in a *Scientist* article titled "In Pursuit of the Longevity Dividend." Decelerating human aging by only seven years "would yield health and longevity benefits greater than what would be achieved with the elimination of cancer or heart disease," they calculated.[85] Clearly, there are great societal benefits to extending the average human health span, but what type of policy changes would need to happen in order to get there faster?

A CHANGE IN POLICY

Almost everyone who looks at how to speed up the pace of longevity research focuses on levels of funding. For instance, out of the NIH budget of around 31 billion in 2009, only 164 million was allocated to research on biological aging.[86] It is time for a reevaluation of priorities in light of how much could be saved if aging were to be delayed even by seven years. Olshansky and his coauthors suggest that the United States should invest $3 billion a year in aging research, which happens to be less than 1 percent of America's Medicare budget. The coalition of longevity scientists call for even more of an investment and urge the international community to get involved as well. Regulatory changes may be necessary, too, because slowing aging is a problem that doesn't fit easily into the Food and Drug Administration's (FDA) go/no-go regulatory calls.

Peter Huber, an analyst at the Manhattan Institute, explains it this way: "all cells, tissues and organs age—and in different ways, at different rates, in different people. As defined by their late-stage clinical symptoms, the diseases of old age are legion. At the FDA they will have to be beaten one at a time or not at all. Which means that nobody is ever going to get 'antiaging' drugs through the FDA as it currently operates."[87] Aging is a whole-body issue, but the FDA has been set up to address specific diseases. The longevity coalition agrees that this is an important problem and suggests that the FDA "be charged with developing new guidelines for testing interventions that do not necessarily target a single specific disease but that retard, arrest, or reverse the structural degeneration and loss of functionality associated with aging."[88] At the very least, then, there are two things the government can do today to help avert the aging crisis and promote longer health spans: change funding priorities in favor of antiaging therapies (which also have the benefit of fighting cancer, heart disease, Alzheimer's, etc. all at once) and change FDA guidelines so that antiaging therapies have real hope for regulatory approval. This last part is especially important because no private firms will fund antiaging research if it is sure to be rejected by the FDA based on how the administrative definitions work.

FIGHTING FOR LIFE AND CHANGING THE WORLD

We are at the cusp of a radical change in social consciousness. Humanity is finally in a position to shed its acceptance of disease and death and instead launch a true offensive against it. That is the good news, but it comes with a qualifier. Great things do not miraculously happen on their own, and health extension is no exception. Some technologists and futurists like to make bold and specific predictions about how many years it will take for human life spans to grow or perhaps even become indefinite. Such posturing might make for exciting headlines, but it can also elicit the opposite result of its intention: that is, if individuals are convinced that the longevity agenda will advance no matter what they do, then they may be inclined to put their efforts elsewhere. Such apathy not only is wrongheaded but also does a disservice to everyone who will suffer and die without the fruits of biotechnical innovation.

The longevity revolution depends on the strong and sustained efforts of a diverse set of people who refuse complacency. Scientists, backed by salespeople, mavens, and connectors, have made great headway in the march toward a brighter future, but it will be realized only when others join them in this cause. Policy makers, activists, journalists, educators, investors, philanthropists, analysts, entrepreneurs, and a whole host of others need to come together to fight for their lives. We now know that aging is plastic and that humanity's time horizons are not set in stone. Larry Ellison, Bill Gates, Peter Thiel, Jeff Bezos, Larry Page, Sergey Brin, and Paul Allen have all recognized the wealth of opportunity in the bioinformatics revolution, but this is not enough. Other heroes must come forward—perhaps there is even one reading this sentence right now.

The goal is more healthy time, which, as we have seen throughout this book, will lead to greater wealth and prospects for happiness. A longer health span means more time to enjoy the wonders of life, including relationships with family and friends, career building, knowledge seeking, adventure, and exploration. It will also include activities that can't be described here because they haven't been invented yet. Just as a family shivering around a fire in 1850 might have had trouble visualizing central heating without smoke, so, too, are there great marvels around the corner that we can't yet imagine. The possibilities, then, are endless but not certain. As science and technology advance, so do our opportunities for eliminating suffering and promoting health and welfare, not only in Western nations but also around the globe. No other mission can be more important.

Notes

CHAPTER 1

1. See the Gerontology Research Group for more on Jeanne Calment: www.grg.org.

2. See S. Jay Olshansky and Bruce A. Carnes, *The Quest for Immortality: Science at the Frontiers of Aging* (New York: Norton, 2001); and David Boyd Haycock, *Mortal Coil: A Short History of Living Longer* (New Haven, CT: Yale University Press, 2008).

3. Haycock, *Mortal Coil*, 21.

4. Lucian Boia, *Forever Young: A Cultural History of Longevity* (London: Reaktion Books, 2004), 60.

5. Haycock, *Mortal Coil*, 22.

6. Ibid., 25.

7. Ibid.

8. William Hansen, *Handbook of Classical Mythology* (Santa Barbara, CA: ABC-CLIO, 2004), 257, 310.

9. Gerald J. Gruman, *A History of Ideas About the Prolongation of Life* (New York: Arno Press, 1977), 43.

10. Ibid.

11. Olshansky and Carnes, *The Quest for Immortality*, 34.

12. George Bernard Shaw, cited in Boia, *Forever Young*, 145.

13. Andrew George, trans., *The Epic of Gilgamesh* (New York: Penguin Classics, 1999). For an online version, see www.ancienttexts.org/library/mesopotamian/gilgamesh/index.html.

14. Haycock, *Mortal Coil*, 169.

15. Tao Tsang, cited in Gruman, *A History of Ideas About the Prolongation of Life*, 45.

16. Oscar Wilde, *The Picture of Dorian Gray*, Project Gutenberg eBook #174, June 9, 2008, www.gutenberg.org/files/174/174-h/174-h.htm.

17. Michael Patrick Gillespie, *The Picture of Dorian Gray: "What the World Thinks Me"* (New York: Twayne, 1995).

18. Ibid.

19. Boia, *Forever Young*, 120.

20. Ibid., 121.

21. Mark Collins Jenkins, "Vampire Forensics: Uncovering the Origins of an Enduring Legend," *National Geographic* 2010, l. 426 Kindle ed.

22. Ruth La Furla, "A Trend with Teeth," *New York Times*, July 1, 2009, www.nytimes.com/2009/07/02/fashion/02VAMPIRES.html.

23. Jenkins, "Vampire Forensics," l. 377.

24. Ibid., l. 386.

25. Mary Wollstonecraft (Godwin) Shelley, *Frankenstein or The Modern Prometheus*, Project Gutenberg eBook #84, June 17, 2008, www.gutenberg.org/files/84/84-h/84-h.htm.

26. Ibid.

27. Carol C. Donley, "Primary Literary Sources on Prolongevity," in *The Fountain of Youth: Cultural, Scientific, and Ethical Perspectives on a Biomedical Goal*, ed. Stephen G. Post and Robert H. Binstock (New York: Oxford University Press, 2004), 438.

28. Jonathan Swift, *Gulliver's Travels into Several Remote Nations of the World*, Project Gutenberg eBook #829, June 15, 2009, chap. 10, www.gutenberg.org/files/829/829-h/829-h.htm.

29. Ibid.

30. Ibid.

31. Haycock, *Mortal Coil*, 86.

32. Hansen, *Handbook of Classical Mythology*, 222.

33. Gruman, *A History of Ideas About the Prolongation of Life*, 12.

34. See memorable quotes from *Bicentennial Man* (1999), www.imdb.com/title/tt0182789/quotes.

35. See www.oscars.org/awards/academyawards/oscarlegacy/1980–1989/58 nominees.html.

36. See memorable quotes from *Cocoon* (1985), www.imdb.com/title/tt0088 933/quotes.

37. Gruman, *A History of Ideas About the Prolongation of Life*, 24.

38. Brandon Keim, "Salamander Discovery Could Lead to Human Limb Regeneration," *Wired News*, July 1, 2009, www.wired.com/wiredscience/2009/07/regeneration/#ixzz0x015ttqG.

39. Olshansky and Carnes, *The Quest for Immortality*, 48.

40. Ibid., 38.

41. Haycock, *Mortal Coil*, 51.

42. Ibid., 54.

43. Ibid., 50.

44. Ibid.,70.

45. Ibid., 28.

46. Boia, *Forever Young*, 74.

47. Haycock, *Mortal Coil*, 30.

48. Ibid., 1–2.

49. Gruman, *A History of Ideas About the Prolongation of Life*, 82.

50. Ibid., 82–83.

51. Ibid., 83.

52. Boia, *Forever Young*, 78.

53. Ibid., 67.

54. Ibid.

55. Mircea Eliade, *Yoga: Immortality and Freedom*, trans. Willard R. Trask (Princeton, NJ: Princeton University Press, 1970), 340

56. Boia, *Forever Young*, 130–133.

57. Review of Books, "The Prolongation of Life," *New York Times*, January 18, 1908, BR25, http://query.nytimes.com/mem/archive-free/pdf?res=9B06E0 DA173EE233A2575BC1A9679C946997D6CF.

58. Boia, *Forever Young*, 135.

59. Haycock, *Mortal Coil*, 175–185.

60. Pope Brock, *Charlatan: America's Most Dangerous Huckster, the Man Who Pursued Him, and the Age of Flimflam* (New York: Three Rivers Press, 2008), 206.

61. Elizabeth Weise, "Stallone Puts Muscle Behind HGH; Raises Alarms," *USA Today*, February 6, 2008, www.usatoday.com/news/health/2008-02-05 -human-growth-hormone_N.htm.

62. Mike Celizic, "Sylvester Stallone Discusses HGH Charge," Todayshow .com, January 18, 2008, http://today.msnbc.msn.com/id/22728530.

63. Suzanne Somers, *Ageless: The Naked Truth About Bioidentical Hormones* (New York: Crown, 2006), 5.

64. William Pepper, *The Medical Side of Benjamin Franklin* (Philadelphia: W. J. Campbell, 1911), 61–62.

65. Neil Ronald Jones, "The Jameson Satellite," Project Gutenberg eBook #26906, October 13, 2008, www.gutenberg.org/files/26906/26906-h/26906-h .htm.

66. Robert C. W. Ettinger, *The Prospect of Immortality* (Garden City, NY: Doubleday, 1965), www.cryonics.org/book1.html.

67. Gregory M Fahy, Brian Wowk et al., "Physical and Biological Aspects of Renal Vitrification," *Organogenesis* 5, no. 3 (July–September 2009): 167–175, www.ncbi.nlm.nih.gov/pmc/articles/PMC2781097/.

CHAPTER 2

1. There is a difference between life span and life expectancy. Life span is how long an individual actually lives. Life expectancy is how long an individual can expect to live, based on averages of the population.

2. Ray Kurzweil, *The Singularity Is Near* (New York: Penguin, 2005), 324.

3. Robert William Fogel, *The Escape from Hunger and Premature Death, 1700–2100* (Cambridge, UK: Cambridge University Press, 2004), 2; Kurzweil, *The Singularity Is Near*, 324.

4. James C. Riley, *Rising Life Expectancy: A Global History* (New York: Cambridge University Press, 2001), 2.

5. Jim Oeppen and James Vaupel, "Broken Limits to Life Expectancy," *Science* 296 (May 10, 2002): 1029.

6. Ibid., supplemental material, table 1.

7. Ibid., 1029.

8. Bruce Grierson, "The Incredible Flying Nonagenarian," *New York Times*, November 25, 2010.

9. National Institute on Aging, "Disability Among Older Americans Continues Significant Decline," December 1, 2006, www.nia.nih.gov/NewsAnd Events/PressReleases/PR20061201DisabilityDecline.htm.

10. Pew Research Center, "Growing Old in America: Expectations vs. Reality," June 29, 2009, http://pewresearch.org/pubs/1269/aging-survey-expectations -versus-reality.

11. Fiona Govan, "First Woman to Have Stem Cell Organ Transplant: Exclusive Interview," *The Telegraph*, November 19, 2008.

12. Paolo Macchiarini, Philipp Jungebluth et al., "Clinical Transplantation of a Tissue-Engineered Airway," *The Lancet* 372, no. 9655 (December 13, 2008): 2023–2030, www.thelancet.com/journals/lancet/article/PIIS0140–6736 (08)61598–6/fulltext. See also Alan Cowell and Denise Grady, "Europeans Announce Pioneering Surgery," *New York Times*, November 20, 2008, www.ny times.com/2008/11/20/health/research/20stemcell.html.

13. Govan, "First Woman to Have Stem Cell Organ Transplant."

14. Cowell and Grady, "Europeans Announce Pioneering Surgery."

15. See www.wfubmc.edu/wfirm/.

16. Wake Forest Medical Center, "Wake Forest Physician Reports First Human Recipients of Laboratory Grown Organs," April 3, 2006, www.wfubmc .edu/AboutUs/NewsArticle.aspx?id=7087.

17. Anthony L. Komaroff, "The Race to Grow New Organs," *Newsweek*, December 7, 2010, www.newsweek.com/2010/12/07/future-of-medicine-growing-new-organs.print.html.

18. See Taylor's lab page: www.stemcell.umn.edu/faculty/Taylor_D/home.html.

19. Miriam Falco, "New Hope May Lie in Lab-Created Heart," CNN, January 14, 2008, http://articles.cnn.com/2008-01-14/health/rebuilt.heart_1_heart-cells-rat-heart-heart-transplants?_s=PM:HEALTH.

20. Thomas H. Petersen, Elizabeth A. Calle et al., "Tissue-Engineered Lungs for in Vivo Implantation," *Science*, July 30, 2010, 538–541.

21. Rachel Bernstein, "Growing Lungs in a Lab: Researchers Move Closer to Goal," *Los Angeles Times*, June 25, 2010, http://articles.latimes.com/2010/jun/25/science/la-sci-lungs-20100625.

22. Jeffrey Kluger, "The 50 Best Inventions of 2010," *Time*, November 11, 2010, www.time.com/time/specials/packages/article/0,28804,2029497_2030617_2029812,00.html.

23. Organovo, "First Fully Bioprinted Blood Vessels," press release, December 8, 2010, www.organovo.com/news/press/42.

24. Ibid.

25. Ann Parson, "A Tissue Engineer Sows Cells and Grows Organs," *New York Times*, July 11, 2006, www.nytimes.com/2006/07/11/health/11prof.html?pagewanted=print.

26. Dr. Badylak has been recognized by the National Institute of Biomedical Imaging and Bioengineering (NIBIB) for his pioneering research in this field. For more, see www.nibib.nih.gov/publicPage.cfm?pageID=665.

27. "A Step Closer to Reversing Type 1 Diabetes," *What's Happening at the McGowan Institute* 8, no. 12 (December 2009), www.mirm.pitt.edu/Newsletter/archive/0912newsletter.asp. See also Katie Falloon, "Patient's Persistence Got Him a New Esophagus at UPMC," *Pittsburgh Post-Gazette*, June 2, 2010, www.post-gazette.com/pg/10153/1062347-114.stm#ixzz18n68rmEU.

28. Elizabeth Cohen, "Woman's Persistence Pays Off in Regenerated Fingertip," CNN, September 9, 2010, www.cnn.com/2010/HEALTH/09/09/pinky.regeneration.surgery/index.html?hpt=C2.

29. AFIRM Wake Forest–Pittsburgh Consortium, "Funding for AFIRM," www.afirmwakepitt.org/About-Us/Funding-for-AFIRM.htm.

30. U.S. Department of Defense, "New Armed Forces Institute of Regenerative Medicine to Lead Way in Caring for Wounded," press release, April 17, 2008, www.defense.gov/reles/release.aspx?releaseid=11842.

31. See "Magic 'Pixie Dust' Made from Pig Bladders Helps 'Regrow' Limbs of Wounded Soldiers," *Daily Mail*, May 5, 2010, www.dailymail.co.uk/sciencetech/article-1270990/Pixie-Dust-pig-bladders-regrows-limbs-wounded-soldiers.html#ixzz18nJxv5m0.

32. See McGowan Institute for Regenerative Medicine, "ECM-Replacement of Lost Muscle Tissue," www.mirm.pitt.edu/programs/clinical_translation/ECM.asp.

33. Morley Safer, "Growing Body Parts," *60 Minutes*, December 13, 2009, www.cbsnews.com/stories/2009/12/11/60minutes/main5968057_page4.shtml ?tag=contentMain;contentBody.

34. Donna Miles, "Regenerative Medicine Shows Promise for Wounded Warriors," American Forces Press Service, February 25, 2010.

35. See DARPA, "Blood Pharming," www.darpa.mil/dso/thrusts/bio/tactbio _med/blood_pharm/index.htm.

36. Katie Drummond, "Darpa's Lab-Grown Blood Starts Pumping," *Wired*, July 9, 2010, www.wired.com/dangerroom/2010/07/darpas-blood-makers-start -pumping/.

37. Eva Szabo, Shravanti Rampalli et al., "Direct Conversion of Human Fibroblasts to Multilineage Blood Progenitors," *Nature* 468 (November 25, 2010), www.nature.com/nature/journal/v468/n7323/full/nature09591.html.

38. McMaster University, "McMaster Scientists Turn Skin into Blood," November 7, 2010, http://fhs.mcmaster.ca/main/news/news_2010/skin_to_blood .html.

39. "Scientists Turn Skin Cells Directly into Blood Cells, Bypassing Middle Pluripotent Step," ScienceDaily, November 8, 2010, www.sciencedaily.com/ releases/2010/11/101107202144.htm.

40. Daniel Schorn, "Scientist Hopes for Stem Cell Success," *60 Minutes*, February 26, 2006, www.cbsnews.com/stories/2006/02/23/60minutes/main134 1635.shtml.

41. Hans S. Keirstead, Gabriel Nistor et al., "Human Embryonic Stem Cell-Derived Oligodendrocyte Progenitor Cell Transplants Remyelinate and Restore Locomotion After Spinal Cord Injury," *Journal of Neuroscience*, May 11, 2005, http://neuro.cjb.net/cgi/content/abstract/25/19/4694.

42. See two of the informative videos here: http://singularityhub.com/2010/ 08/02/gerons-embryonic-stem-cell-clinical-trials-for-spinal-cord-injury-have -returned/.

43. David Wright and Dan Childs, "Medical Milestone: Genetics Company Begins First Embryonic Stem-Cell Treatment on Patient," ABC News, October 11, 2010, http://abcnews.go.com/print?id=11853497. See also Geron, "Geron Initiates Clinical Trial of Human Embryonic Stem Cell-Based Therapy," October 11, 2010, www.geron.com/media/pressview.aspx?id=1235.

44. National Institutes of Health, "Stem Cells and Diseases," http://stem-cells.nih.gov/info/health.asp.

45. Paolo Rama, M.D., Stanislav Matuska, M.D. et al., "Limbal Stem-Cell Therapy and Long-Term Corneal Regeneration," *New England Journal of Medicine*, July 8, 2010, http://www.nejm.org/doi/full/10.1056/NEJMoa0905955.

46. See www.tcacellulartherapy.com/fda_clinical_trials.html; and www.cytori .com/Innovations/ClinicalTrials/HeartDisease.aspx.

47. See www.regenexx.com/.

48. Regenexx, "Regenerative-Science FAQ," www.regenexx.com/wp-content/ uploads/2010/08/Regenerative-Science-FAQs-8.21.10.pdf (last accessed January 11, 2011).

49. "Jarvis Green Gets Contract with Houston Texans, Attributes It to Regenexx Stem Cell Injections," *Regenerative Sciences*, December 15, 2010, www.regenexx.com/2010/12/jarvis-green-gets-contract-with-houston-texans -attributes-it-to-regenexx-stem-cell-injections/.

50. Phone conversation with Jarvis Green. January 13, 2011.

51. "Regenerative-Science FAQ."

52. FDA, "Regenerative Sciences, Inc.," July 25, 2008, www.fda.gov/Biologics BloodVaccines/GuidanceComplianceRegulatoryInformation/Compliance Activities/Enforcement/UntitledLetters/ucm091991.htm; FDA, "FDA Seeks Injunction Against Colorado Manufacturer of Cultured Cell Product," August 6, 2010, www.fda.gov/NewsEvents/Newsroom/PressAnnouncements/ucm221 656.htm.

53. Dr. Katherine High of the Children's Hospital of Philadelphia explains that the "key to safety is careful animal studies, careful dose escalation, and attention to safety signals." Phone interview, March 8, 2011.

54. "One Shot of Gene Therapy and Children with Congenital Blindness Can Now See," Children's Hospital of Philadelphia, October 24, 2009, http:// multivu.prnewswire.com/mnr/chop/40752/; Francesca Simonelli, Albert M. Maguire et al., "Gene Therapy for Leber's Congenital Amaurosis Is Safe and Effective Through 1.5 Years After Vector Administration," *Molecular Therapy*, December 2009, www.nature.com/mt/journal/v18/n3/full/mt2009277a.html.

55. "Gene Therapy Helps Blind Boy See," CBS News, October 26, 2009, www.cbsnews.com/stories/2009/10/26/earlyshow/health/main5421926.shtml. For a video of Corey and the surgeons who treated him, see www.youtube.com/ watch?v=H0RvTOF1fEc.

56. Alessandro Aiuti, M.D., Ph.D., Federica Cattaneo, M.D. et al., "Gene Therapy for Immunodeficiency Due to Adenosine Deaminase Deficiency," *New England Journal of Medicine*, January 29, 2009, www.nejm.org/doi/full/10.1056/ NEJMoa0805817.

57. Christine Lagorio, "Gene Therapy Breakthrough, First Documented Cases of Gene Altering Save 2 Melanoma Patients," CBS News, August 31, 2006, www .cbsnews.com/stories/2006/08/31/health/main1955526.shtml?tag=content Main;contentBody.

58. John King and Dr. Sanjay Gupta, "Cancer Researcher: 'This Is Just a Start,'" CNN, August 31, 2006, http://articles.cnn.com/2006–0831/health/

cnna.rosenberg_1_attack-tumors-cancer-researcher-colon-cancer?_s=PM :HEALTH.

59. Nicholas Wade, "In New Way to Edit DNA, Hope for Treating Disease," *New York Times*, December 28, 2009, www.nytimes.com/2009/12/29/health/research/29zinc.html.

60. See www.sangamo.com/index.php.

61. Sangamo BioSciences, "Sangamo BioSciences Announces Presentation of Preliminary Data from Phase 1 Safety Trial of SB-728-T for HIV/AIDS," January 19, 2010, http://investor.sangamo.com/releasedetail.cfm?ReleaseID =438350.

62. "Bone Marrow Cures HIV Patient," BBC News, November 13, 2008. See also Elizabeth Landau and Miriam Falco, "Why HIV Advance Is Not a Universal Cure," CNN Health, December 15, 2010, http://pagingdrgupta .blogs.cnn.com/2010/12/15/why-hiv-advance-is-not-a-universal-cure/.

63. Cynthia Kenyon, J. Chang et al., "C. Elegans Mutant That Lives Twice as Long as Wild Type," *Nature* 366 (1993): 461–464.

64. Cynthia Kenyon, "The Plasticity of Aging: Insights from Long-Lived Mutants," *Cell* 120 (February 25, 2005): 449–460.

65. Cynthia Kenyon, "From Worms to Mammals: Genes That Control the Rate of Aging," NIH director's Wednesday afternoon lecture series, Bethesda, Maryland, 2008, http://videocast.nih.gov/Summary.asp?File=14308.

66. Alex Crevar, "As the Worm Turns," *Georgia Magazine* (University of Georgia), 2004, http://www.uga.edu/gm/604/FeatWorm.html.

67. Srinivas Ayyadevara, Ramani Alla et al., "Remarkable Longevity and Stress Resistance of Nematode PI3K-Null Mutants," *Aging Cell* (2007), www .uams.edu/update/news/aging_cell.pdf.

68. Antonia Tomas-Loba, Ignacio Flores et al., "Telomerase Reverse Transcriptase Delays Aging in Cancer-Resistant Mice," *Cell*, September 2008.

69. Joseph A. Baur, Kevin J. Pearson et al., "Resveratrol Improves Health and Survival of Mice on a High-Calorie Diet," *Nature* 444 (November 16, 2006), www.nature.com/nature/journal/v444/n7117/abs/nature05354.html.

70. David Stipp, *The Youth Pill: Scientists on the Brink of an Anti-Aging Revolution* (New York: Penguin, 2010), 3–4.

71. Ricki J. Colman, Rozalyn M. Anderson et al., "Caloric Restriction Delays Disease Onset and Mortality in Rhesus Monkeys," *Science* 325 (July 10, 2009), www.ncbi.nlm.nih.gov/pmc/articles/PMC2812811/.

72. See www.sirtrispharma.com/pipeline.html.

73. Michael Rae, "NIA's ITP Confirms: Resveratrol Does Not Extend Lifespan; Limited Benefit to Rapamycin," SENS Foundation, October 27, 2010, www.sens.org/node/1759.

74. Michael Mason, "One for the Ages: A Prescription That May Extend Life," *New York Times*, October 31, 2006, www.nytimes.com/2006/10/31/health/nutrition/31agin.html?pagewanted=1&_r=1.

75. David E. Harrison, Randy Strong et al., "Rapamycin Fed Late in Life Extends Lifespan in Genetically Heterogeneous Mice," *Nature* 460 (July 16, 2009), www.nature.com/nature/journal/v460/n7253/full/nature08221.html.

76. Claudia Dreifus, "Finding Clues to Aging in the Fraying Tips of Chromosomes," *New York Times*, July 3, 2007, www.nytimes.com/2007/07/03/science/03conv.html.

77. Calvin B. Harley, Weimin Liu et al., "A Natural Product Telomerase Activator as Part of a Health Maintenance Program," *Rejuvenation Research*, September 7, 2010, www.liebertonline.com/doi/full/10.1089/rej.2010.1085.

78. Chris Woolston, "Pricey Telomerase Supplements, Touted as Longevity Boosters, Are Unproven," *Los Angeles Times*, December 20, 2010, www.latimes.com/health/la-he-skeptic-telomeres-20101220,0,6925196,print.story.

79. See www.tasciences.com/ta-65/.

80. "Genome Announcement a Milestone, but Only a Beginning," CNN, June 26, 2000, http://archives.cnn.com/2000/HEALTH/06/26/human.genome.05/index.html.

81. Epigenetics is one of these new discoveries. See Brandon Keim, "Early Reports from the 'Dark Matter' of the Genome," *Wired News*, December 22, 2010, www.wired.com/wiredscience/2010/12/genomic-dark-matter/.

82. John Lauerman, "Complete Genomics Drives Down Cost of Genome Sequence to $5,000," Bloomberg News, February 5, 2009, www.bloomberg.com/apps/news?pid=newsarchive&refer=home&sid=aEUlnq6ltPpQ.

83. "Your Genome in Minutes: New Technology Could Slash Sequencing Time," ScienceDaily, December 31, 2010, www.sciencedaily.com/releases/2010/12/101220121111.htm.

84. Francis Collins, "A Genome Story: 10th Anniversary Commentary," Scientific American, June 25, 2010, www.scientificamerican.com/blog/post.cfm?id=a-genome-story-10th-anniversary-com-2010-06-25.

85. Boston University School of Medicine, New England Centenarian Study, "Why Study Centenarians? An Overview," www.bumc.bu.edu/centenarian/overview/.

86. Albert Einstein College of Medicine, "Einstein Launches SuperAgers.com to Spotlight Aging Research," November 1, 2010, www.einstein.yu.edu/home/news.asp?ID=582.

87. J. Craig Venter Institute, "First Self-Replicating Synthetic Bacterial Cell," www.jcvi.org/cms/research/projects/first-self-replicating-synthetic-bacterial-cell/overview/.

88. Katie Drummond, "Pentagon Looks to Breed Immortal 'Synthetic Organisms,' Molecular Kill-Switch Included," *Wired News*, February 5, 2010, www.wired.com/dangerroom/2010/02/pentagon-looks-to-breed-immortal-synthetic-organisms-molecular-kill-switch-included/.

89. Aubrey de Grey with Michael Rae, *Ending Aging: The Rejuvenation Breakthroughs That Could Reverse Human Aging in Our Lifetime* (New York: St. Martin's Press, 2007).

90. Jason Pontin, "The SENS Challenge," *MIT Technology Review*, July 28, 2005, www.technologyreview.com/blog/pontin/14968/.

91. SENS Foundation, "Research Themes."

CHAPTER 3

1. Interview with Michael O'Connor, July 17, 2009.

2. Harry Cline, "There Is More to GPS Tractors Than Straight Lines," *Western Farm Press*, June 2000, www.novariant.com/news/pdfs/autofarm_feature_stories/0600WesternFarmPressMoreToGPS.pdf.

3. Interview with O'Connor. He has since left the company and was replaced as CEO by Chris Ragot. See www.novariant.com/news/articles/0806 2010_newceo.cfm.

4. See tomato example on the AutoFarm Web site: www.gpsfarm.com/SpecialtyCropGrower/tabid/77/Default.aspx.

5. Geoff Colvin, "Food for Thought," *Fortune*, June 17, 2008, http://money.cnn.com/2008/06/16/magazines/fortune/colvin_deere.fortune/index.htm.

6. U.S. Census Bureau, "History 1800 and Profile of General Demographic Characteristics: 2000," www.census.gov/history/www/through_the_decades/fast_facts/1800_fast_facts.html; U.S. Census Bureau, "Population Clocks, World POPClock," www.census.gov/main/www/popclock.html.

7. U.S. Census Bureau, Population Division, "Historical Estimates of World Population," www.census.gov/ipc/www/worldhis.html; U.S. Census Bureau, "Population Clocks, World POPClock."

8. Leonid Gavrilov and Natalia Gavrilova, "Demographic Consequences of Defeating Aging," *Rejuvenation Research* 13, nos. 2–3 (2010).

9. U.S. Census Bureau, International Database, "World Population Growth Rate," June 2009 update, www.census.gov/ipc/www/idb/worldgrgraph.php.

10. Paul Hofheinz, "Gates on Technology, AIDS, and Why Malthus Was Wrong," ZDNet, January 29, 2001, www.zdnet.com/news/gates-on-technology-aids-and-why-malthus-was-wrong/113884.

11. Mikko Myrskylä, Hans-Peter Kohler, and Francesco C. Billari, "Advances in Development Reverse Fertility Declines," *Nature* 460 (August 6, 2009): 741–743, www.nature.com/nature/journal/v460/n7256/abs/nature08230.html.

12. United Nations, Department of Social and Economic Affairs, Population Division, "World Population to 2300," 2004, www.un.org/esa/population/publications/longrange2/WorldPop2300final.pdf.

13. Thomas Malthus, *An Essay on the Principle of Population* (1798), Library of Economics and Liberty, www.econlib.org/library/Malthus/malPop1.html #I.17.

14. Paul Ehrlich, *The Population Bomb* (New York: Ballantine Books, 1968), prologue.

15. Bjorn Lomborg, *The Skeptical Environmentalist: Measuring the Real State of the World* (Cambridge, UK: Cambridge University Press, 2001), 61–62.

16. Ed Regis, "The Doomslayer," *Wired*, February 1997, 12, www.wired.com/wired/archive/5.02/ffsimon_pr.html.

17. Ibid.

18. These were chromium, copper, nickel, tin, and tungsten.

19. Jennifer Clapp and Peter Dauvergne, *Paths to a Green World: The Political Economy of the Global Environment* (Cambridge, MA: MIT Press, 2005), 103.

20. David McClintick and Ross B. Emmett, "Betting on the Wealth of Nature: The Simon-Ehrlich Wager," *PERC Reports* 23, no. 3 (September 2005), www.perc.org/articles/article588.php.

21. UN Department of Economic and Social Affairs, Population Division, "The World at Six Billion," October 12, 1999, www.un.org/esa/population/publications/sixbillion/sixbillion.htm.

22. John Tierney, "Betting the Planet," *New York Times Magazine*, December 2, 1990, 52, www.nytimes.com/1990/12/02/magazine/betting-on-the-planet .html?scp=1&sq=John%20Tierney&pagewanted=print.

23. National Research Council, Working Group on Population Growth and Economic Development, Committee on Population, *Population Growth and Economic Development: Policy Questions* (Washington, DC: National Academies Press, 1986), 16–17.

24. Samuel H. Preston, "The Effect of Population Growth on Environmental Quality," *Population Research and Policy Review* 15 (April 1996): 96.

25. Hofheinz, "Gates on Technology."

26. For more on the Mensa organization, see www.mensa.org/index0.php ?page=10.

27. "The Wonder Wire," *Globe and Mail*, August 18, 1989.

28. American Council on Science and Health, "Dr. Norman Borlaug, Who Saved a Billion Lives, Honored by Congress This Week," July 16, 2007, www .acsh.org/factsfears/newsID.991/news_detail.asp.

29. Henry I. Miller, "More Crop for the Drop," *Los Angeles Times*, April 27, 2009, www.latimes.com/news/opinion/commentary/la-oe-miller27-2009apr27 ,0,3682826.story.

30. Saline conditions can refer to the water or to the soil. According to Dr. Amy Kaleita of Iowa State University, "Saline conditions in agricultural environments today are common in arid regions where water in the soil evaporates quickly, leaving trace salts behind that build up over time. These are usually counteracted by applying even more water than plants require, the extra water being used to flush salts out of the root zone. So salt-tolerant crops will require less irrigation—thus it's simultaneously a quality and quantity issue." E-mail interview, September 2, 2009.

31. University of California, Davis, "Genetically Engineered Tomato Plant Grows in Salty Water," press release, July 25, 2001, www.news.ucdavis.edu/search/news_detail.lasso?id=5840.

32. See "Drought-Tolerant Wheat: 'Promising Results,'" GMO Safety, August 2008, www.gmo-safety.eu/en/news/654.docu.html.

33. Martin LaMonica, "IBM Plunges into the 'Smart Grid for Water,'" Cnet News, September 4, 2009, http://news.cnet.com/8301-11128_3-10345122 -54.html?tag=newsCategoryArea.1.

34. Peter Huber, "Wealth Is Green," Speakout.com, March 23, 2000, http:// speakout.com/activism/opinions/5039-1.html.

35. Don Coursey, "The Demand for Environmental Quality," University of Chicago, December 1992, as discussed in Matthew Brown and Jane S. Shaw, "Prosperity and Environment: Does Prosperity Protect The Environment?" PERC Reports 17, no. 1 (February 1999), www.perc.org/articles/article357.php ?view=print.

36. Gene M. Grossman and Alan B. Krueger, "Environmental Impact of a North American Free Trade Agreement," Working Paper 3914 (Cambridge, MA: National Bureau of Economic Research, November 1991).

37. Gene Grossman and Alan B. Krueger, "Economic Growth and the Environment," Quarterly Journal of Economics 110, no. 2 (May 1995): 353–377, www.jstor.org/pss/2118443.

38. Ibid.

39. Kuheli Dutt, "Governance, Institutions, and the Environment-Income Relationship: A Cross-Country Study," Environment, Development, and Sustainability, December 12, 2007, www.springerlink.com/content/661x3u658wk81507/.

40. Indeed, in 2007 the U.S. Supreme Court ordered the Environmental Protection Agency (EPA) to determine whether CO_2 posed a threat to Americans, and in 2009 the EPA declared that carbon dioxide and five other greenhouse gasses endanger human health. This opens the door to greater government regulations. U.S. per capita personal income can be found at the U.S. Department of Commerce, Bureau of Economic Analysis, www.bea.gov/regional/reis/default .cfm?selTable=CA1–3&section=2. For a summary of President Obama's energy

plan, see "Energy and the Environment," www.whitehouse.gov/agenda/energy_and_environment/.

41. Carl Safina, cited in "Environmental Values," *The Economist*, April 13, 2009, www.economist.com/world/international/displaystory.cfm?story_id=13474652.

42. Bill Clinton, "Protecting Our Environment and Public Health," speech, January 11, 2000, http://clinton4.nara.gov/WH/Accomplishments/environment.html.

43. Bruce Yandle, Madhusudan Bhattarai, and Maya Vijayaraghavan, "Environmental Kuznets Curves: A Review of Findings, Methods, and Policy Implications," Research Study 02-1 (Bozeman, MT: PERC, April 2004), www.perc.org/pdf/rs02_1a.pdf.

44. Per capita income numbers come from the 2007 World Bank Report, World Development Indicators database, December 15, 2010, http://siteresources.worldbank.org/DATASTATISTICS/Resources/GNIPC.pdf. Life expectancy numbers come from the World Health Organization, www.who.int/whosis/whostat2007_1mortality.pdf.

45. "Down in the Dumps: Managing Waste Properly Is Expensive, Which Is Why Rich Countries Mostly Do It Better Than Poor Ones," *The Economist*, February 28, 2009, 5.

46. Ibid.

47. Ibid.

48. Ibid.

49. According to Diane Katz, director of risk, environment, and energy policy studies at the Vancouver-based Fraser Institute, humans are already turning their waste into energy. In an email interview September 3, 2009, she said, "Landfill methane is commonly used to generate power. Some cities burn household trash to generate electricity. Biomass (dead trees, branches and tree stumps, yard clippings and wood chips) are also burned as fuel."

50. See Carl Zimmer, "Scientist of the Year: Jay Keasling," *Discover*, December 2006, http://discovermagazine.com/2006/dec/cover; and Biotechnology Industry Organization, "Jay Keasling Receives Inaugural Biotech Humanitarian Award," May 2009, www.bio.org/news/pressreleases/newsitem.asp?id=2009_0520_02.

51. For an entertaining and informative discussion with Jay Keasling, see this video from the March 10, 2009, episode of *The Colbert Report*: www.colbertnation.com/the-colbert-report-videos/221178/march-10-2009/jay-keasling.

52. Synthetic Genomics, "Synthetic Genomics Inc and ExxonMobil Research and Engineering Company Sign Exclusive, Multi-year Agreement to Develop Next Generation Biofuels Using Photosynthetic Algae," press release, July 14, 2009, www.syntheticgenomics.com/media/press/71409.html.

53. Jad Mouawad, "Exxon to Invest Millions to Make Fuel from Algae," *New York Times,* July 13, 2009, www.nytimes.com/2009/07/14/business/energy-environment/14fuel.html?_r=1&scp=2&sq=biofuel%20drop%20in%20bucket&st=cse.

54. Katie Howell, "Plant-Derived Fuels Could Be Certified for Flights Within a Year, Says Boeing Exec," *New York Times,* May 29, 2009, www.nytimes.com/gwire/2009/05/29/29greenwire-plant-derived-fuels-could-be-certified-for-fli-24118.html.

55. "60 Minutes Video: Cold Fusion Is Hot Again," CNet News, April 20, 2009, http://news.cnet.com/8301-11386_3-10223427–76.html?tag=mncol.

56. Analytical chemist Pamela Mosier-Boss of the U.S. Navy's Space and Naval Warfare Systems Center released a peer-reviewed report on "the production of highly energetic neutrons from a LENR device." LENR means low energy nuclear reaction, a euphemism that has been adopted because the words "cold fusion" tend to be very controversial. See David Hambling, "Navy Scientists Zip Lips on Cold Fusion Tests," *Wired News,* March 26, 2009, www.wired.com/dangerroom/2009/03/navy-scientists/.

57. Ray Kurzweil, cited in Natasha Lomas, "Nanotech to Solve Global Warming by 2028," IT Pro, November 20, 2008, http://management.silicon.com/itpro/0,39024675,39345604,00.htm.

58. Robin Lloyd, "Solar Power to Rule in 20 Years, Futurists Say," LiveScience, February 19, 2008, www.livescience.com/environment/080219-kurzweil-solar.html.

59. For a detailed discussion of how nanotechnology could be used to extend life, see Robert A. Freitas Jr., "Comprehensive Nanorobotic Control of Human Morbidity and Aging," in *The Future of Aging: Pathways to Human Life Extension,* ed. Gregory M. Fahy, Michael D. West, L. Stephen Coles, and Steven B. Harris (New York: Springer, 2010), pp. 685–805.

60. Prachi Patel, "Nano Sponge for Oil Spills," *MIT Technology Review,* June 2, 2008, www.technologyreview.com/nanotech/20846/.

61. "First Generation Prototype," SeaSwarm, 2010, http://senseable.mit.edu/seaswarm/ss_prototype.html.

62. Bill Joy, "Why the Future Doesn't Need Us," *Wired,* April 2000, www.wired.com/wired/archive/8.04/joy_pr.html. The idea that nanobots will get out of control and consume all of the earth's biomass is often referred to as the "gray goo" problem.

63. *The Charlie Rose Show,* November 26, 2002, www.michaelcrichton.net/video-charlierose-11-26-02.html.

64. See Bill McKibben, *Enough: Staying Human in an Engineered Age* (New York: Henry Holt, 2003).

65. For more on issue self-replicating technology, or the "gray goo" problem, see Robert A. Freitas Jr., "Some Limits to Global Ecophagy by Biovorous Nanoreplicators, with Public Policy Recommendations," April 2000, www .rfreitas.com/Nano/Ecophagy.htm.

66. Abby Frank, "Nanotechnology Myths," EarthSky, 2004, www.earthsky .org/article/nanotechnology-myths.

67. "No Small Matter! Nanotech Particles Penetrate Living Cells and Accumulate in Animal Organs," ETC Group, no. 76 (May–June 2002), www.etcgroup .org/en/materials/publications.html?pub_id=192.

68. Craig A. Poland, Rodger Duffin, Ian Kinloch, Andrew Maynard, William A. H. Wallace, Anthony Seaton, Vicki Stone, Simon Brown, William MacNee, and Ken Donaldson, "Carbon Nanotubes Introduced into the Abdominal Cavity of Mice Show Asbestos-Like Pathogenicity in a Pilot Study," *Nature Nanotechnology* 3 (2008): 423–428, www.nature.com/nnano/journal/v3/n7/abs/ nnano.2008.111.html.

69. Fred Krupp and Chad Holliday, "Let's Get Nanotech Right," *Wall Street Journal*, June 14, 2005, www.edf.org/documents/5177_OpEd_WSJ050614.pdf.

70. "Environmental Defense–DuPont Nano Risk Framework," February 26, 2007, www.edf.org/documents/5989_Nano%20Risk%20Framework-final%20 draft-26feb07-pdf.pdf.

71. ETC Group, "Broad International Coalition Issues Urgent Call for Strong Oversight of Nanotechnology," press release, July 31, 2007, www.etcgroup.org/ en/materials/publications.html?pub_id=651.

72. Chris Phoenix and Mike Treder, "Applying the Precautionary Principle to Nanotechnology," Center for Responsible Nanotechnology, January 2004, www.crnano.org/precautionary.htm.

73. Ray Kurzweil, "Nanotechnology Dangers and Defenses," *Nanotechnology Perceptions: A Review of Ultraprecision Engineering and Nanotechnology* 2, no. 1 (March 27, 2006), www.kurzweilai.net/meme/frame.html?main=/articles/art 0653.html.

CHAPTER 4

1. Ellen Goodman, "A Wide Gulf Between Cures and 'Perfection,'" *Sun Sentinel*, January 25, 2002, http://articles.sun-sentinel.com/2002-01-25/news/ 0201240945_1_bioethics-total-ban-embryos.

2. Leon R. Kass, "Why Not Immortality?" in *The Future Is Now: America Confronts the New Genetics*, ed. William Kristol and Eric Cohen (Lanham, MD: Rowman and Littlefield, 2002).

3. Ibid., 325.

4. Bill McKibben, "Mr. Natural," *Outside,* May 2003, http://outside.away
.com/outside/bodywork/200305/200305_mr_natural_1.html.

5. Ibid.

6. Arthur Caplan, "Good, Better, or Best?" in *Human Enhancement,* ed. Julian Savulescu and Nick Bostrom (New York: Oxford University Press, 2009), 202.

7. Kass, "Why Not Immortality?" 326.

8. See www.clintonbushhaitifund.org/.

9. Kass, "Why Not Immortality?" 327.

10. Daniel Callahan, cited in Christine Overall, *Aging, Death, and Human Longevity: A Philosophical Inquiry* (Berkeley and Los Angeles: University of California Press, 2003), 39–40.

11. Kass, "Why Not Immortality?" 327.

12. For an excellent discussion of both positive and negative fictional characters who live a long time, see Joseph D. Miller, "Living Forever or Dying in the Attempt: Mortality and Immortality in Science and Science Fiction," in *Immortal Engines,* ed. George Slusser, Gary Westfahl, and Eric S. Rabkin (Athens: University of Georgia Press, 1996), 77–89.

13. John Harris, *Enhancing Evolution: The Ethical Case for Making Better People* (Princeton, NJ: Princeton University Press, 2007), 60.

14. Kass, "Why Not Immortality?" 328.

15. John Harris, "Enhancements Are a Moral Obligation," in *Human Enhancement,* ed. Savulescu and Bostrom, 131.

16. C. A. J. Coady, "Playing God," in *Human Enhancement,* ed. Savulescu and Bostrom, 164.

17. James M. Pethokoukis, "Bioethicist William Hurlbut on the Dangers of Radical Lifespan Extension," *U.S. News and World Report,* May 28, 2004, www
.usnews.com/usnews/tech/nextnews/archive/next040528.htm.

18. Ramez Naam, *More Than Human* (New York: Broadway Books, 2005), 31.

19. Tim Cavanaugh, "Wake Me Up When Men Get Pregnant: Biological Transhumanism Starts the 21st Century on the Wrong Foot," *Reason,* March 2010.

20. Alexandra Minna Stern and Howard Markel, "The History of Vaccines and Immunization: Familiar Patterns, New Challenges," *Health Affairs* 24, no. 3 (2005), http://content.healthaffairs.org/cgi/content/full/24/3/611.

21. Julie Steenhuysen and Bill Berkrot, "Drug Fights Tumors in Advanced Lung Cancer," Reuters, June 5, 2010, www.reuters.com/article/idUSN051596 2620100605?type=marketsNews.

22. "Gene Therapy Helps Blind Boy See," CBS News, October 26, 2009, www.cbsnews.com/stories/2009/10/26/earlyshow/health/main5421926.shtml.

For a video of Corey and the surgeons who treated him, see www.youtube.com/watch?v=H0RvTOF1fEc.

23. C. Ben Mitchell and C. Christopher Hook, "State-Sponsored Liberal Eugenics Has Just Begun," Institute of Biotechnology and the Human Future, 2006, www.thehumanfuture.org/commentaries/eugenics/eugenics_commentary _cbmitchell01.html.

24. Johann Hari, "Why I Support Liberal Eugenics," *The Independent*, July 6, 2006, www.independent.co.uk/opinion/commentators/johann-hari/johann-hari -why-i-support-liberal-eugenics-406804.html.

25. Naam, *More Than Human*, 166–167.

26. Ronald Bailey, *Liberation Biology: The Scientific and Moral Case for the Biotech Revolution* (New York: Prometheus Books, 2005), 180.

27. Ronald Dworkin, *Sovereign Virtue* (Cambridge, MA: Harvard University Press, 2000), 452.

28. Michael Sandel, *The Case Against Perfection* (Cambridge, MA: Harvard University Press, 2007), 83.

29. Michael Sandel, "The Case Against Perfection," *The Atlantic*, April 2004.

30. Frances Kamm, "What Is and Is Not Wrong with Enhancement," in *Human Enhancement*, ed. Savulescu and Bostrom, 123–124.

31. Audrey R. Chapman, "The Social and Justice Implications of Extending the Human Lifespan," in *The Fountain of Youth: Cultural, Scientific, and Ethical Perspectives on a Biomedical Goal*, ed. Stephen G. Post and Robert H. Binstock (New York: Oxford University Press, 2004), 353.

32. Nick Bostrom, "Recent Developments in the Ethics, Science, and Politics of Life-Extension," *Aging Horizons* 3 (Autumn–Winter 2005): 28–34, www.fhi.ox.ac.uk/__data/assets/pdf_file/0004/5926/life-extension.pdf.

33. Ibid.

34. Jonathan Weiner, *Long for This World* (New York: HarperCollins, 2010), 261.

35. Francis Fukuyama, *Our Posthuman Future: Consequences of the Biotechnology Revolution* (New York: Picador, 2002), 172.

36. George Annas, "Genism, Racism, and the Prospect of Genetic Genocide," The Future of Human Nature: A Symposium on the Promises and Challenges of the Revolutions in Genomics and Computer Science, Pardee Center Conference Series, Boston University, Boston, Massachusetts, April 2003.

37. Fukuyama, *Our Posthuman Future*, 171, 175.

38. Annas, "Genism."

39. C. J. L. Murray, S. C. Kulkarni, C. Michaud, N. Tomijima, M. T. Bulzacchelli et al., "Eight Americas: Investigating Mortality Disparities Across Races, Counties, and Race-Counties in the United States," *PLoS Med* 3, no. 9 (2006), www.plosmedicine.org/article/info:doi/10.1371/journal.pmed.0030260.

40. Fukuyama, *Our Posthuman Future*, 158.

41. Christine Overall, "Life Enhancement Technologies: The Significance of Social Category Membership," in *Human Enhancement*, ed. Savulescu and Bostrom, 331.

42. Ibid., 339.

43. James Hughes, *Citizen Cyborg* (Boulder, CO: Westview Press, 2004), 233.

44. Michael Cox and Richard Alm, *Myths of Rich and Poor* (New York: Basic Books, 1999), 161–163.

45. Comments on Andrew Hessel's Web page, http://openwetware.org/wiki/Andrew_Hessel (last accessed July 9, 2010).

46. The $199 price for 23andMe's service requires a $5 per month subscription to the company's personal genome service. This is far less expensive than the $1,000 the company charged for the service in 2007.

47. Ray Kurzweil, *The Singularity Is Near* (New York: Penguin, 2005), 95.

48. Ray Kurzweil, cited in Alan Boyle, "Reaching for Immortality," MSNBC .com, July 15, 2010, http://cosmiclog.msnbc.msn.com/_news/2010/07/15/468 5717-reaching-for-immortality.

49. Kurzweil, *The Singularity Is Near*, 41.

50. Ibid.

51. Scott E. Page, *The Difference: How the Power of Diversity Creates Better Groups, Firms, Schools, and Societies* (Princeton, NJ: Princeton University Press, 2007).

52. Cox and Alm, *Myths of Rich and Poor*, 49.

53. Romer's ideas are widely discussed, but perhaps the most interesting current summary can be found in Sebastian Mallaby, "The Politically Incorrect Guide to Ending Poverty," *The Atlantic*, July–August 2010, www.theatlantic.com/magazine/print/2010/07/the-politically-incorrect-guide-to-ending-poverty/8134/.

54. Matt Ridley, *The Rational Optimist: How Prosperity Evolves* (New York: HarperCollins, 2010), 352.

55. Ibid., 14–15.

56. Ronald Bailey, "Post-Scarcity Prophet," *Reason*, December 2001, http://reason.com/archives/2001/12/01/post-scarcity-prophet/1.

57. Max More, "The Myth of Stagnation," in *Death and Anti-death*, ed. Charles Tandy, vol. 7 (Palo Alto, CA: Ria University Press, 2010), www.maxmore.com/mythofstagnation.htm.

CHAPTER 5

1. Rahul Bedi and Kate Devlin, "Indian Woman Has First Child at Age of 70," *The Telegraph*, December 8, 2008, www.telegraph.co.uk/news/worldnews/asia/india/3684395/Indian-woman-has-first-child-at-age-of-70.html.

2. Lisa Belkin, "70-Year-Old Woman Gives Birth," *New York Times*, December 9, 2008, http://parenting.blogs.nytimes.com/2008/12/09/pregnant-at-70/.

3. William Saletan, "Motherhood at 70: Meet the World's Newest Oldest Mom," *Slate*, December 9, 2008, www.slate.com/id/2206334/.

4. Andy Beckett, "Time, Gentlemen," *The Age*, May 8, 2006, www.theage .com.au/news/in-depth/time-gentlemen/2006/05/07/1146940408372.html.

5. Lawrence M. Hinman, "Are Some Parents Too Old? Age Restrictions in Postmenopausal Pregnancies and Adoptions," University of San Diego, http://ethics.sandiego.edu/LMH/Papers/Papers/Older_Pregnancies.html.

6. Daniel Woolls, "Oldest Woman to Give Birth Dies, Leaving Twins," Associated Press, July 15, 2009, www.daytondailynews.com/news/nation-world -news/oldest-woman-to-give-birth-dies-leaving-twins-205743.html.

7. Ibid.

8. It is worth remembering that female fertility into the mid-forties is not a recent phenomenon and has been more common than is frequently recognized. There is evidence that female fertility rates at the population level can be relatively high into the forties and that in some cases these rates have remained relatively static at least over the last sixty years. The four European Union countries (France, Scotland, Ireland, and Italy) where birth rates to the over forties are more than 4 percent of live births are also countries with a large Catholic population, some of whom may follow the church's prohibition on the use of contraception. As an example, in Scotland around 4.5 percent of all births are to women aged forty and older, and this has remained constant from the 1950s to today. In countries such as Canada the trend until recently has been the reverse, with a drop from 3.1 percent in 1951 to around 1.4 percent in 1991. Female fertility over forty declined from the 1950s to the 1990s as a result of access to contraception ("the pill" hit the market in the 1960s). See European Commission, Health and Consumer Protection Directorate-General, Table C2, Life Births by Mother's Age at Last Birthday, http://ec.europa.eu/health/ph_information/dissemination/echi/echi_03_en.pdf; Table 3.1, Live Births, Numbers and Percentages, by Age of Mother and Marital Status of Parents, www.gro-scotland.gov.uk/files1/stats/07t3 -1.pdf; Table B1, Maternal Age Data, www.statcan.gc.ca/pub/11-516-x/sectionb/ 4147437-eng.htm#B1_14; and Live Births by Age of Mother, CanSim, Statistics Canada database, http://cansim2.statcan.gc.ca/.

9. David Rapp, "America's First Test-Tube Baby Turns 25," *American Heritage*, December 28, 2006, www.americanheritage.com/articles/web/20061228 -in-vitro-fertilization-reproductive-technology-ivf-elizabeth-carr-howard-jones -georgeanna-jones.shtml.

10. Chana Gazit and Hilary Klotz Steinman, "Test Tube Babies," American Experience, PBS, October 23, 2006, www.pbs.org/wgbh/americanexperience/ features/introduction/babies-introduction/.

11. See "Infertility Advances at the Jones Institute," www.jonesinstitute.org/ivf-jones.html.

12. Elizabeth Carr, "Lives: Grandmother of Thousands," *New York Times*, December 25, 2005, www.nytimes.com/2005/12/25/magazine/25lives.html

13. Centers for Disease Control and Prevention, *Assisted Reproductive Technology Success Rates* (Washington, DC: GPO, 1996 and 2006), 1, 13, respectively, www.cdc.gov/art/ARTReports.htm.

14. Centers for Disease Control and Prevention, *Assisted Reproductive Technology Success Rates*, 2006 ed., 11; Centers for Disease Control and Prevention, *Assisted Reproductive Technology Success Rates*, 1996 ed., 6, www.cdc.gov/art/ARTReports.htm.

15. Rob Stein, "In Vitro Fertilization Can't Reverse Aging's Effects," *Washington Post*, January 15, 2009.

16. Centers for Disease Control and Prevention, *Assisted Reproductive Technology Success Rates*, 2006 ed., 26, Figure 14, www.cdc.gov/ART/ART2006/508PDF/2006ART.pdf.

17. Centers for Disease Control and Prevention, *Assisted Reproductive Technology Success Rates*, 2006 ed., 57, Figure 45, www.cdc.gov/ART/ART2006/508PDF/2006ART.pdf.

18. Colorado Center for Reproductive Medicine, "Egg Freezing Now Available as Clinical Treatment," August 17, 2009, www.colocrm.com/EggFreezingNowAvailableAsClinicalTreatment.pdf.

19. Sarah-Kate Templeton, "Revealed: First Ovary Transplant Baby," *Sunday Times* (London), November 9, 2008.

20. Kristina Fiore, "Woman Has Second Baby After Ovarian Tissue Transplant," ABC News, February 24, 2010, http://abcnews.go.com/Health/WellnessNews/ovarian-tissue-transplant-leads-birth-time/story?id=9929965.

21. Erik Ernst, Stinne Bergholdt et al. "The First Woman to Give Birth to Two Children Following Transplantation of Frozen/Thawed Ovarian Tissue," *Human Reproduction* 25, no. 5 (January 25, 2010): 1280–1281, http://humrep.oxfordjournals.org/content/25/5/1280.abstract.

22. Centers for Disease Control and Prevention, "Delayed Childbearing: More Women Are Having Their First Child Later in Life," NCHS Data Brief, No. 16 (Washington, DC: GPO, 2009), 1, www.cdc.gov/nchs/data/databriefs/db21.pdf.

23. Ibid.

24. Exceptions to the doubling rule are Japan, where overall there was a decline in the total birthrate, and France, where the 1991 birthrate of women over forty was already relatively high. CDC Vital Statistics, "Demographic Characteristics of Mother," http://205.207.175.93/VitalStats/ReportFolders/ReportFolders.aspx. The UK data include Scotland. Additional information is from Table 3.1,

Live Births, Numbers, and Percentages, by Age of Mother and Marital Status of Parents, www.gro-scotland.gov.uk/files1/stats/07t3-1.pdf. Data for England and Wales are from Table 4.1, Age of Women at Conception, www.statistics.gov.uk/STATBASE/ssdataset.asp?vlnk=9558. Data for Japan, France, and Germany are all taken from UN Demographic Statistics: 1991 data are from Table 6:6, Live Births by Age of Mother and Live-Birth Order; 1990–1998 data are from http://unstats.un.org/unsd/demographic/products/dyb/DYBNat/NatStatTab06.pdf; and 2006 data are from the UN Demographic Yearbook, Table 10, Live Births by Age of Mother, Sex of the Child and Urban/Rural Residence: Latest Available Year, 1997–2006, http://unstats.un.org/unsd/demographic/products/dyb/default.htm.

25. Hadley Leggett, "A Fertility First: Human Egg Cells Grow Up in Lab," *Wired News*, July 14, 2009, www.wired.com/wiredscience/2009/07/humanegg/.

26. Min Xu, Susan L. Barrett, Erin West-Farrell, Laxmi A. Kondapalli, Sarah E. Kiesewetter, Lonnie D. Shea, and Teresa K. Woodruff, "In Vitro Grown Human Ovarian Follicles from Cancer Patients Support Oocyte Growth," *Human Reproduction*, July 13, 2009, http://humrep.oxfordjournals.org/cgi/content/abstract/24/10/2531.

27. Leggett, "A Fertility First."

28. Lisa Belkin, "Your Old Man," *New York Times*, April 1, 2009, www.nytimes.com/2009/04/05/magazine/05wwln-lede-t.html?_r=1&ref=health.

29. Alice Park, "Scientists Create Human Sperm from Stem Cells," Time.com, July 8, 2009, www.time.com/time/health/article/0,8599,1909164,00.html.

30. U.S. Census Bureau, "Families and Living Arrangements," 2008, www.census.gov/population/www/socdemo/hh-fam.html (chart link: MS2).

31. U.S. Department of Labor, Quick Stats 2007, www.dol.gov/wb/stats/main.htm.

32. Ibid. For historical data, see Susan E. Shank, "Women and the Labor Market: The Link Grows Stronger," *Monthly Labor Review* 111 (1988).

33. Mark Regnerus, "Say Yes. What Are You Waiting For?" *Washington Post*, April 26, 2009, www.washingtonpost.com/wp-dyn/content/article/2009/04/24/AR2009042402122.html.

34. Ibid.

35. Maria Kefalas, Frank Furstenberg, and Laura Napolitano, "Marriage Is More Than Being Together: The Meaning of Marriage Among Young Adults in the United States," MacArthur Foundation Network on Transitions to Adulthood Working Paper, September 2005, www.transad.pop.upenn.edu/downloads/kefalasmarriagenorms.pdf.

36. "Does Marriage Still Matter? Talking with Young Adults About Marriage and Relationships," Qualitative Study: Coming of Age in America, MacArthur Foundation Network on Transitions to Adulthood, January 2007, www.transad.pop.upenn.edu/downloads/doesmarriagestillmatter.pdf.

37. Kefalas, Furstenberg, and Napolitano, "Marriage Is More Than Being Together."

38. Ibid.

39. David Popenoe, "Cohabitation, Marriage, and Child Wellbeing: A Cross-National Perspective," National Marriage Project, Rutgers University, 2008, http://marriage.rutgers.edu/Publications/NMP2008CohabitationReport.pdf.

40. Paul Taylor, Cary Funk, and April Clark, "Generation Gap in Values, Behaviors: As Marriage and Parenthood Drift Apart, Public Is Concerned About Social Impact," Pew Research Center, July 1, 2007, http://pewresearch .org/assets/social/pdf/Marriage.pdf.

41. Peg Tyre, "Bringing Up Adultolescents: Millions of Americans in Their 20s and 30s Are Still Supported by Their Parents. The Me Generation Is Raising the Mini-Me Generation," *Newsweek*, March 25, 2002, http://www.newsweek .com/id/153586; Linda Perlman Gordon and Susan Morris Shaffer, *Mom, Can I Move Back in with You?: A Survival Guide for Parents of Twentysomethings* (New York: Penguin, April 2004).

42. Jeffrey Jensen Arnett, cited in Christina Ianzito, "Full House: When Kids Move Back Home Parents Struggle with Adult Children's Return," *Washington Post*, November 16, 2004.

43. Helen Fisher, *Anatomy of Love: A Natural History of Mating, Marriage, and Why We Stray* (New York Random House, 1992), 113.

44. Ibid.

45. Anushka Asthana and Denis Campbell, "US Study Says Divorce Is Linked to Age and Education," *The Observer*, September 27, 2009, www.guardian .co.uk/lifeandstyle/2009/sep/27/divorce-linked-to-age-education.

46. Frank F. Furstenberg, Rubén G. Rumbaut, and Richard A. Settersten, "On the Frontier of Adulthood: Emerging Themes and New Directions," MacArthur Foundation Network on Transitions to Adulthood Policy Brief, no. 1, October 2004, www.transad.pop.upenn.edu/downloads/ch1-fff-formatted.pdf.

47. Ethan Watters, *Urban Tribes: Are Friends the New Family?* (London: Bloomsbury, 2004), 30.

48. Ibid., 185.

49. William A. Sadler, *The Third Age: Six Principles for Personal Growth and Rejuvenation After Forty* (New York: Da Capo Press, 2001).

50. Center for Third Age Leadership, "What Is the Third Age?" www.third agecenter.com/whatis3rdage.htm (last accessed November 17, 2009).

51. Jan Erik Kristiansen, "Age Differences at Marriage: The Times They Are a Changing." Statistics Norway, January 31, 2005, www.ssb.no/english/magazine/ art-2005-01-31-01-en.html.

52. Ibid.

53. New Jersey Department of Health and Senior Services, "Marriages and Divorces," 2003, www.state.nj.us/health/chs/stats03/marriage.shtml.

54. Ruth Houston, "Extreme Age Differences in Marriage Can Lead to Infidelity," Authorsden.com, May 25, 2004, www.authorsden.com/visit/viewArticle .asp?id=14130.

55. Dan Jewel, "But Who's Counting: Age Defying Duos," *People* 52, no. 14 (October 11, 1999), www.people.com/people/archive/article/0,,20129448,00.html.

56. Shripad D. Tuljapurkar, Cedric O. Puleston, and Michael D. Gurven, "Why Men Matter: Mating Patterns Drive Evolution of Human Lifespan," *PLoS ONE* 2, no. 8 (2007): e785, www.ncbi.nlm.nih.gov/pmc/articles/PMC 1949148/?tool=pubmed.

57. Miller McPherson, Lynn Smith-Lovin, and James M Cook, "Birds of a Feather: Homophily in Social Networks," *Annual Review of Sociology* 27 (August 2001): 415–444.

58. Elizabeth Taylor was married eight times to seven husbands. For a complete listing, see http://en.wikipedia.org/wiki/Elizabeth_Taylor#Marriages.

59. Meredith Small, "The Perfect Family Is a Myth," LiveScience, December 5, 2008, www.livescience.com/culture/081205-hn-family.html.

60. Lawrence M. Hinman, "Are Some Parents Too Old? Age Restrictions in Postmenopausal Pregnancies and Adoptions," Paper published online, University of San Diego, http://ethics.sandiego.edu/LMH/Papers/Papers/Older _Pregnancies.html.

61. Nancy Recker, "In Praise of Older Parents," Ohio State University, 2007, http://ohioline.osu.edu/hyg-fact/5000/pdf/Older_Parents.pdf.

62. Ronit Baras, "What Is the Right Age Gap for Siblings to Have Good Relationship?" http://ezinearticles.com/?What-is-the-Right-Age-Gap-For-Siblings -to-Have-Good-Relationship?&id=1788855.

63. Alex Cutting, "Family and Child Development: Siblings," BBC Open University, May 1, 2006, www.open2.net/healtheducation/family_childdevelopment/ siblings.html.

64. Nina Howe and Holly Recchia, "Sibling Relations and Their Impact on Children's Development," in *Encyclopedia on Early Childhood Development* (Montreal: Centre for Research in Human Development, Concordia University, April 2006), www.enfant-encyclopedie.com/Pages/PDF/Howe-RecchiaANGxp.pdf.

65. Jan Kok and Hilde Bras, "Clustering and Dispersal of Siblings in the North-Holland Countryside, 1850–1940," *Historical Social Research* 33, no. 3 (2008). www.virtualknowledgestudio.nl/staff/jan-kok/clustering-kok-bras2008.pdf.

66. Pnina S. Klein, Ruth Feldman, and Shlomit Zarur, "Mediation in a Sibling Context: The Relations of Older Siblings' Mediating Behaviour and Younger Siblings' Task Performance," *Infant and Child Development*, no. 11 (2002): 321–333.

67. Rupert Brown, Group Processes, 2nd ed. (Oxford, UK: Blackwell, 2002), 41–356. A good discussion of Henri Tajfel's social identity theory can be found in Roger Brown, *Social Psychology* (New York: Macmillan, 1986), 584–585.

68. McPherson, Smith-Lovin, and Cook, "Birds of a Feather."

69. A good general discussion of this phenomenon can be found in Martha Augoustinos and Iain Walker, *Social Cognition* (London: Sage, 2006). Of particular interest are chapter 3, on the essentials of attribution theory, and chapter 9, which applies this to understanding how we interpret both our own groups and others.

70. Ian Rankin, *A Question of Blood* (London: Orion Books, 2003), 284–285.

71. Peter Carruthers, "Multiple Memory Systems," in *The Architecture of the Mind*, ed. Peter Carruthers (Oxford, UK: Blackwell, 2006), 120–130.

72. E. Tory Higgins, "Saying-Is-Believing Effects: When Sharing Reality About Something Biases Knowledge and Evaluation," in *Shared Cognition in Organizations*, ed. Leigh T. Thompson, John M. Levine, and David M. Messick (Mahwah, NJ: Laurence Erlbaum, 1999), 44.

73. Ute Schönpflug, "Intergenerational Transmission of Values: The Role of Transmission Belts," *Journal of Cross-Cultural Psychology* 32 (2001): 174.

74. GDP per capita is based on a model developed by Angus Maddison to facilitate cross-country comparisons. See Angus Maddison, *The World Economy* (Paris: OECD, 2003). Birthrates are derived from UN data, Table, Total Fertility (children per women), http://data.un.org/Browse.aspx?d=POP.

75. Aubrey de Grey, "What Is Human Nature?" Big Think interview, December 17, 2007, http://bigthink.com/ideas/4432.

76. www.childfree.net/ (last accessed February 2, 2010).

77. Brenda McEvoy DeVellis, Barbara Strudler Wallston, and David Acker, "Childfree by Choice: Attitudes and Adjustment of Sterilized Women," *Population and Environment* 7, no. 3 (September 1984).

78. U.S. Department of Commerce, Economics and Statistics Administration, "Fertility of American Women: 2006," August 2008, www.census.gov/prod/2008pubs/p20-558.pdf.

79. Centers for Disease Control and Prevention/National Center for Health Statistics, "Fertility, Family Planning, and Women's Health: New Data from the 1995 National Survey of Family Growth" Series 23, no. 19 (May 1997), www.cdc.gov/nchs/data/series/sr_23/sr23_019.pdf; Centers for Disease Control and Prevention/National Center for Health Statistics, "Fertility, Family Planning, and Reproductive Health of U.S. Women: Data from the 2002 National Survey of Family Growth" Series 23, no. 5 (December 2005), www.cdc.gov/nchs/nsfg/abc_list_c.htm#childlessness.

80. Mikko Myrskylä, Hans-Peter Kohler, and Francesco C. Billari, "Advances in Development Reverse Fertility Declines," *Nature* 460 (August 6,

2009): 741–743, www.nature.com/nature/journal/v460/n7256//full/nature08 230.html#B4.

81. Stephanie Coontz, *Marriage, a History: From Obedience to Intimacy or How Love Conquered Marriage* (New York: Viking, 2005).

82. Ibid.

83. Cheryl Elman and Andrew S. London, "Sociohistorical and Demographic Perspectives on U.S. Remarriage in 1910," *Social Science History* 26, no. 1 (Spring 2002): 201–202.

84. Ibid.

85. "Inheritance and Property," in *Encyclopedia of Children and Childhood in Society*, www.faqs.org/childhood/In-Ke/Inheritance-and-Property.html.

86. Australian Bureau of Statistics, "Family Formation: Remarriage Trends of Divorced People," Australian Social Trends, 1999, www.abs.gov.au/ausstats/abs@.NSF/2f762f95845417aeca25706c00834efa/a9b78b550e8d5e77ca2570ec00111f19!OpenDocument.

87. Joan D. Atwood, "10 Necessary Steps to Stepfamily Integration," *Marriage and Family Living* (1990): 20–25.

88. Froma Walsh, *Normal Family Processes* (New York: Guilford Press, 2003).

89. S. Golombok, C. Murray, P. Brinsden, and H. Abdalla, "Social Versus Biological Parenting: Family Functioning and the Socio-emotional Development of Children Conceived by Egg or Sperm Donation," *Journal of Child Psychology and Psychiatry* 40, no. 4 (1999): 519–527.

90. Katrina Clark, "My Father Was an Anonymous Sperm Donor," *Washington Post*, December 17, 2006, www.washingtonpost.com/wp-dyn/content/article/2006/12/15/AR2006121501820.html.

91. S. Golombok, F. MacCallum, and E. Goodman, "The 'Test-Tube' Generation: Parent-Child Relationships and the Psychological Well-Being of IVF Children at Adolescence," *Child Development* 72, no. 2 (2001): 599–608.

CHAPTER 6

1. Bob Shallit, "At 92, a Real Estate Go-Getter; Agent Virginia Raskin Is Not Slowing Down, Racking Up Sales in a Down Market," *Sacramento Bee*, June 21, 2008, D1.

2. John P. Robinson and Geoffrey Godbey, *Time for Life: The Surprising Ways Americans Use Their Time* (University Park: Pennsylvania State University Press, 1997).

3. John P. Robinson, "Americans' Use of Time Project Survey" (Ann Arbor: University of Michigan, 1971).

4. Pew Research Center, "Who's Feeling Rushed? (Hint: Ask a Working Mom)" (Washington, DC: Pew Research Center Publications, February 2006).

5. Gary Becker, "A Theory of the Allocation of Time," *The Economic Journal* 75, no. 299 (September 1965): 503.

6. Staffan B. Linder, *The Harried Leisure Class* (New York: Columbia University Press, 1970).

7. Elizabeth Arias, United States Life Tables 2004, National Vital Statistics Reports, Table 12, December 28, 2007, 34, www.cdc.gov/nchs/data/nvsr/nvsr56/nvsr56_09.pdf.

8. Julian Simon, *The State of Humanity* (Malden, MA: Blackwell, 1998), 27.

9. David E. Bloom and David Canning, "The Health and Wealth of Nations," *Science* 287 (February 18, 2000), www.sciencemag.org/content/287/5456/1207.full.

10. Even a 0.1 percent increase in real per capita income growth would be valuable and would have a huge impact over time.

11. S. Jay Olshansky, Daniel Perry, Richard A. Miller, and Robert N. Butler, "In Pursuit of the Longevity Dividend," *The Scientist*, March 2006, 28–36.

12. S. Jay Olshansky, "A Wrinkle in Time: A Modest Proposal to Slow Aging and Extend Healthy Life," *Slate*, November 12, 2010, www.slate.com/id/2274468/pagenum/all/#p2.

13. Kevin M. Murphy and Robert H. Topel, "The Value of Health and Longevity," *Journal of Political Economy* 114 (2006): 872.

14. Ibid.

15. Gary Becker, Tomas J. Philipson, and Rodrigo R. Soares, "The Quantity and Quality of Life and the Evolution of World Inequality," Paper no. 9765 (Cambridge, MA: National Bureau of Economic Research, June 2003).

16. Gary Becker, cited in "The Upside of Globalization: Longevity Gains in Developing Countries," Capital Ideas, University of Chicago, February 2006, www.chicagobooth.edu/capideas/feb06/2.aspx.

17. Education does not automatically guarantee an increase in productivity. There are some economists who have argued that one of the purposes of education is for job-seekers to obtain "signals" that are used by employers to determine aptitude and ability. For more, see Michael Spence, "Job Market Signaling," *Quarterly Journal of Economics* 87, no. 3 (August 1973): 355–374. Likewise, not all useful education is in the form of traditional education.

18. Rodolfo E. Manuelli and Ananth Seshadri, "Human Capital and the Wealth of Nations," 2005 Meeting Papers, No. 56 (Storrs, CT: Society for Economic Dynamics, May 2005), 35.

19. Diane Ravitch, "American Traditions of Education," in *A Primer on America's Schools*, ed. Terry Moe (Stanford, CA: Hoover Institution Press, 2001), 13.

20. See www.waitingforsuperman.com.

21. Howard Gardner, *Five Minds for the Future* (Boston: Harvard Business School Publishing, 2006).

22. Jordan Kaplan, cited in Stephanie Armour, "Generation Y: They've Arrived at Work with a New Attitude," *USA Today*, November 6, 2005, www.usatoday.com/money/workplace/2005-11-06-gen-y_x.htm.

23. Riaz Hassan, "Social Consequences of Manufactured Longevity," *MJA* 173 (2000): 601–603 (Adelaide, South Australia: Flinders University).

24. Clayton M. Christensen, Michael B. Horn, and Curtis W. Johnson, *Disrupting Class: How Disruptive Innovation Will Change the Way the World Learns* (New York: McGraw-Hill, 2008), 100.

25. Tom Lowry, "Extreme Experience," *BusinessWeek*, August 28, 2008, www.businessweek.com/magazine/content/08_36/b4098046922925.htm?campaign_id=rss_daily.

26. Jim Oeppen and James Vaupel, "Broken Limits to Life Expectancy," *Science* 296 (May 10, 2002), supplemental material, table 2.

27. Christopher F. Chabris, David I. Laibson, and Jonathon P. Schuldt, "Intertemporal Choice," in *The New Palgrave Dictionary of Economics*, 2nd ed. (London: Palgrave Macmillan, 2007).

28. Lowry, "Extreme Experience."

29. Phone interview with Donald Boudreaux, June 23, 2008.

30. Simona Cremante, *Leonardo da Vinci: Artist, Scientist, Inventor* (Milan: Guinti Editore, 2008); A. Haase, Gottfried Landwehr, and Eberhard Umbach, *Röntgen Centennial: X-Rays in Natural and Life Sciences* (Hackensack, NJ: World Scientific Publishing, 1997), 3.

31. Walter Isaacson, *A Benjamin Franklin Reader* (New York: Simon and Schuster, 2005).

32. Richard A. Posner, *Aging and Old Age* (Chicago: University of Chicago Press, 1995), 167.

33. Ker Than, "The Psychological Strain of Living Forever," LiveScience, May 24, 2006, www.livescience.com/health/060524_immortality_psychology.html.

34. U.S. Department of Labor, Bureau of Labor Statistics, "Time Use on an Average Work Day for Employed Persons Ages 25–54 with Children," American Time Use Survey, 2009, http://www.bls.gov/tus/charts/.

35. Robinson and Godbey, *Time for Life*, 96.

36. Doug Moore, "More Workers Shun Retirement, Stay on the Job," *St. Louis Post Dispatch*, November 23, 2008, www.stltoday.com/stltoday/news/stories.nsf/stlouiscitycounty/story/CD464BFEF223B8B1862575090014D4D5?OpenDocument.

37. Already social security in the United States is unsustainable. See Stephen Ohlemacher, "Social Security Fund Slides into Permanent Deficit," Associated Press, January 27, 2011, www.usatoday.com/money/economy/2011-01-27-social-security_N.htm.

38. Interestingly, President Roosevelt proposed the act as a more moderate version of a popular program that Californian Francis Townsend was proposing, which would have made retirement mandatory at age sixty and offered generous pensions of up to $200 a month, an amount equivalent at the time to a full salary for a middle-income worker. See Mary-Lou Weisman, "The History of Retirement, from Early Man to A.A.R.P.," *New York Times*, March 21, 1999, http://query.nytimes.com/gst/fullpage.html?res=9E0CE3D8103EF932 A15750C0A96F958260.

39. Jon Gertner, "Are You Ready for 100? By the Middle of the Century Between 800,000 and 4 Million Americans Will Be Older Than 100. What Will That Mean for You?" CNN Money.com, http://money.cnn.com/magazines/moneymag/moneymag_archive/2001/04/01/299317/index.htm.

40. Ibid.

41. Gillian Leithman, "The Psychology of Saving," Ezine Articles, http://ezinearticles.com/?The-Psychology-of-Saving&id=1224522.

42. Karl-Erik Warneryd, *The Psychology of Saving: A Study on Economic Psychology* (Northampton, MA: Edward Elgar, 1999), 111.

43. Some may argue that a strong faith in medical technology could drastically reduce savings because individuals might think they would be able to simply work all their lives and therefore would see no need to save for any retirement. This might be the response of some but seems unlikely for the majority because a longer life would mean a greater potential for financial hiccups that would require savings, not to mention that many would save to finance extra education.

44. Warneryd, *The Psychology of Saving*, 309.

45. Ibid.

46. The "Freedom 55" campaign by the London Life Insurance Company was an example of what we might see more of in the future. See www.freedom 55financial.com/freedom55/english/default.asp.

47. Alicia H. Munnell, Anthony Webb et al., "Inheritance and Wealth Transfer to Baby Boomers" (New York: MetLife Mature Market Institute, December 2010), 2.

48. Bob Morris, "Stop Spending My Inheritance," *New York Times*, July 30, 2006, www.nytimes.com/2006/07/30/fashion/sundaystyles/30AGE.html.

49. Geoff Gloeckler, "Jack Welch Launches Online MBA," *BusinessWeek*, June 22, 2009. See also www.jwmi.com/.

CHAPTER 7

1. Extensive research conducted by Jewish studies professor Alan Segal makes it clear that every single human culture has created an idea of what

happens to us after we die. See Alan Segal, *Life After Death: A History of the Afterlife in Western Religion* (New York: Doubleday Religion, 2004).

2. Ernest Becker, *The Denial of Death* (New York: Simon & Schuster, 1973).

3. Daniel Schorn, "The Quest For Immortality," *60 Minutes*, January 1, 2006, www.cbsnews.com/stories/2005/12/28/60minutes/main1168852.shtml.

4. "How to Live Forever: Abolishing Ageing," *The Economist*, January 3, 2008, www.economist.com/node/10423439.

5. Rabbi Elliot N. Dorff, "Becoming Yet More Like God: A Jewish Perspective on Radical Life Extension," in *Religion and the Implications of Radical Life Extension*, ed. Derek F. Maher and Calvin Mercer (New York: Palgrave Macmillan, 2009), 69.

6. Sherry E. Fohr, "Karma, Austerity, and Time Cycles: Jainism and Radical Life Extension," in *Religion and the Implications of Radical Life Extension*, ed. Maher and Mercer, 82. Jainism is an Indian religion that teaches nonviolence and austerity.

7. Ronald Cole-Turner, "Extreme Longevity Research: A Progressive Protestant Perspective," in *Religion and the Implications of Radical Life Extension*, ed. Maher and Mercer, 59.

8. Ibid., 60.

9. Phone interview with Lawrence Iannaccone, April 1, 2010.

10. Peter Berger, "Epistemological Modesty: An Interview with Peter Berger," *Christian Century*, October 29, 1997, 972–978.

11. Carl Sagan, *The Varieties of Scientific Experience: A Personal View of the Search for God*, ed. Ann Druyan (New York: Penguin, 2006), 64.

12. "God: After a Lengthy Career, the Almighty Recently Passed into History. Or Did He?" *The Economist*, December 23, 1999, www.economist.com/node/347578.

13. "Epistemological Modesty: An Interview with Peter Berger," *Christian Century*, October 29, 1997, www.religion-online.org/showarticle.asp?title=240.

14. Charles T. Mathewes, "An Interview with Peter Berger," *Hedgehog Review*, Spring and Summer 2006, 152.

15. Phone interview with Todd Johnson, February 8, 2011.

16. Pippa Norris and Ronald Inglehart, *Sacred and Secular: Reexamining the Secularization Thesis* (New York: Cambridge University Press, 2004), 5. According to Bran Grim, a senior researcher in religion at the Pew Forum, religion has grown owing to the collapse of communism as well as the strong growth in Asia, Africa, and Latin America. Phone interview with Bran Grim, April 21, 2010.

17. Recent data from the Pew Foundation show that 83 percent of Americans say they are affiliated with a religion. See Pew Forum on Religion and Public Life, "US Religious Landscape Survey: Religious Affiliation: Diverse and

Dynamic," February 2008, http://religions.pewforum.org/pdf/report-religious
-landscape-study-full.pdf.

18. Andrew M. Greeley and Michael Hout, "Americans' Increasing Belief in Life After Death: Religious Competition and Acculturation," *American Sociological Review* 64, no. 6 (December 1999): 813.

19. Ibid.

20. For more on the economics of religion, see Lawrence R. Iannaccone, "Introduction to the Economics of Religion," *Journal of Economic Literature* 36 (September 1998): 1465–1496, www.religionomics.com/iannaccone/papers/Iannaccone%20-%20Introduction%20to%20the%20Economics%20of%20Religion.pdf.

21. Greeley and Hout, "Americans' Increasing Belief in Life After Death," 832.

22. "O Come All Ye Faithful," *The Economist*, November 1, 2007, www.economist.com/node/10015239.

23. Todd M. Johnson and Brian J. Grim, "International Religious Demography: An Overview of Sources and Methodology," in *Oxford Handbook of the Economics of Religion*, ed. Rachel M. McCleary (Oxford, UK: Oxford University Press, 2011), 374.

24. Norris and Inglehart, *Sacred and Secular*.

25. Ibid, 108.

26. "Kentucky Creation Museum Draws Crowds Along with Controversy," *USA Today*, July 23, 2007, www.usatoday.com/travel/news/2007-07-23-creation-museum-attendance_N.htm.

27. John Micklethwait and Adrian Wooldridge, *God Is Back: How the Global Revival of Faith Is Changing the World* (New York: Penguin, 2010), 18.

28. Ibid., 4–8.

29. Phone interview with Iannaccone.

30. Agence-France Press, "Students Flock to Study Creationism at University," March 8, 2010, www.clipsyndicate.com/video/play/1342650.

31. See Phil Zuckerman, "Atheism, Secularity, and Well-Being: How the Findings of Social Science Counter Negative Stereotypes and Assumptions," *Sociology Compass*, 2009, 952, www.pitzer.edu/academics/faculty/zuckerman/Zuckerman_on_Atheism.pdf.

32. Darren Sherkat, "Religion and Higher Education: The Good, the Bad, and the Ugly," Social Science Research Council Online Forum, February 6, 2007, http://religion.ssrc.org/reforum/Sherkat.pdf.

33. Ibid.

34. Pew Forum on Religion and Public Life, "Educational Level by Religious Tradition," U.S. Religious Landscape Survey, 2008, http://religions.pewforum.org/pdf/table-education-by-tradition.pdf.

35. Sherkat, "Religion and Higher Education," 3.

36. Francis Collins, *The Language of God: A Scientist Presents Evidence for Belief* (New York: Simon and Schuster, 2006), 166.

37. Ibid., 200.

38. Pew Forum on Religion and Public Life, "Faith in Flux: Changes in Religious Affiliation in the United States," April 27, 2009, http://pewforum.org/docs/?DocID=409.

39. Ibid.

40. Ibid.

41. Luis Lugo, cited in David A. Patten, "Study: Half of All Americans Switch Religions," Newsmax.com, May 1, 2009, http://newsmax.com/Newsfront/americans-religion-change/2009/05/01/id/329840.

42. Ralph Wood, Peter Hill, and Bernard Spilka, *The Psychology of Religion*, 4th ed. (New York: Guilford Press, 2009), 356.

43. Norris and Inglehart, *Sacred and Secular*.

44. Nicholas Kristof, "God and Evolution," *New York Times*, February 12, 2005, www.nytimes.com/2005/02/12/opinion/12kristof.html?_r=2.

45. Edward O. Wilson, *On Human Nature* (Cambridge, MA: Harvard University Press, 1978).

46. Edward O. Wilson, *Consilience: The Unity of Knowledge* (New York: Vintage Books, 1998), 270.

47. Dean H. Hamer, *The God Gene: How Faith Is Hardwired into Our Genes* (New York: Doubleday, 2004).

48. Wood, Hill, and Spilka, *The Psychology of Religion*, 62–66.

49. Dinesh D'Souza, *Life After Death: The Evidence* (Washington, DC: Regnery, 2009), 44.

50. Phone interview with William Swing, February 4, 2010.

51. Ibid.

52. Fohr, "Karma, Austerity, and Time Cycles," 79.

53. Ibid., 82. *Ayus* karma is "life" karma, which determines life span.

54. Ibid.

55. Dorff, "Becoming Yet More Like God," 72.

56. Ibid.

57. Nigel M. de S. Cameron and Amy Michelle DeBaets, "Be Careful What You Wish For? Radical Life Extension Coram De: A Reformed Protestant Perspective," in *Religion and the Implications of Radical Life Extension*, ed. Maher and Mercer, 44.

58. Ghulam Ahmed Parvez, cited in Aisha Y. Musa, "A Thousand Years, Less Fifty: Toward a Quranic View of Extreme Longevity," in *Religion and the Implications of Radical Life Extension*, ed. Maher and Mercer, 127–128.

59. Musa, "A Thousand Years, Less Fifty," 128.

60. Livia Kohn, "Told You So: Extreme Longevity and Daoist Realization," in *Religion and the Implications of Radical Life Extension*, ed. Maher and Mercer, 87.

61. Ibid., 95.

62. Ibid., 96.

63. Ibid.

64. Lawrence R. Iannaccone, "Why Strict Churches Are Strong," *American Journal of Sociology* 99, no. 5 (March 1994): 1180.

65. Ibid., 1183.

66. Gary Laderman, *Sacred Matters: Celebrity Worship, Sexual Ecstasies, the Living Dead, and Other Signs of Religious Life in the United States* (New York: New Press, 2009), xiv.

67. Ibid., xiv.

68. Ibid., xv.

69. Ibid., 79.

70. Ibid.

71. Gary Laderman, "Sacred and Profane: The 'Cult' of Oprah Inflames Religious Right," Religion Dispatches blog, April 27, 2008, www.religiondispatches .org/archive/mediaculture/200/sacred%26profane:_the_"cult"_of_oprah _inflames_religious_right. The YouTube video about Oprah can be found at www.youtube.com/watch?v=JW4LLwkgmqA.

72. Laderman, *Sacred Matters*, 79.

73. I am friends with many prominent transhumanists, and many of them are not religious about it but are simply working to make sure technology is implemented in a way that best benefits society. Indeed, while writing this book, I served on the board of directors of Humanity Plus and I also helped to start Singularity University, based at NASA, which focuses on exploring exponentially growing technology and how it can benefit the world. For more information, see http://humanityplus.org/; and http://singularityu.org/. I do not consider my involvement with these organizations to be religious, but I have met many people in the movement whose actions fit within Laderman's definition.

74. E-mail interview with Calvin Mercer, March 22, 2009.

75. Ray Kurzweil, *The Singularity Is Near* (New York: Penguin, 2005), 374.

76. Ibid., 374–375.

77. Ibid., 371.

78. Ibid., 7.

79. Ibid., 5.

80. Ibid., 372.

81. Ibid., 375.

82. Ray Kurzweil and Terry Grossman, *Transcend: Nine Steps to Living Well Forever* (New York: Rodale Books, 2009).

83. Kurzweil, *The Singularity Is Near*, 390.

84. Memebox, "Ray Kurzweil: The Singularity Is Not a Religion," October 27, 2008, www.youtube.com/watch?v=CLy0tTfw8i0&feature=player_embedded.

85. Kurzweil, *The Singularity Is Near*, 370.

86. Ibid., 389.

CHAPTER 8

1. Sanjay Gupta, *Chasing Life* (New York: Warner Wellness, 2007), 236.

2. Ibid.

3. Malcolm Gladwell, *The Tipping Point* (New York: Little, Brown, 2000), 70–86.

4. *The Oprah Show*, June 30, 2009, www.oprah.com/health/David-Murdocks -Diet-and-Fitness-Routine-Video.

5. Dr. Mehmet Oz, "The Benefits of Calorie Restriction," *The Oprah Show*, June 30, 2009, www.oprah.com/health/Dr-Oz-on-Living-Longer-with-a-Calorie -Restriction-Diet/1.

6. Ibid.

7. Dr. Mehmet Oz, "High-Tech Ways to Extend Your Life," *The Oprah Show*, March 24, 2009, www.oprah.com/health/Life-Extension-Technology-and-Tissue -Regeneration.

8. Ibid.

9. Gladwell, *The Tipping Point*, 66.

10. Aubrey de Grey with Michael Rae, *Ending Aging: The Rejuvenation Break-throughs That Could Reverse Human Aging in Our Lifetime* (New York: St. Martin's Press, 2007), 10.

11. Aubrey de Grey, *The Mitochondrial Free Radical Theory of Aging* (Austin, TX: Landes Bioscience, November 2003); Michael Finkel, "Life Begins at 140," *GQ*, May 2010.

12. Interview with Aubrey de Grey, November 20, 2010.

13. Finkel, "Life Begins at 140."

14. Ben Goertzel, "AI Against Aging: Accelerating the Quest for Longevity via Intelligent Software," Biomind LLC, www.biomind.com/AI_Against_Aging.pdf.

15. Ibid.

16. Ibid.

17. See Ray Kurzweil's biography, www.singularity.com/fullbiography.html.

18. Ray Kurzweil, *The Singularity Is Near* (New York: Penguin, 2005), 323.

19. Ray Kurzweil and Terry Grossman, *Fantastic Voyage: Live Long Enough to Live Forever* (New York: Plume, 2005). They also published a similar book in 2009 titled *Transcend: Nine Steps to Living Well Forever* (New York: Rodale Books, 2009). See also www.rayandterry.com/index.asp.

20. For more information, see http://singularityu.org. I am an associate founder of Singularity University and am currently a member of the Board of Trustees.

21. The tracks policy, law, and ethics; and finance and entrepreneurship are also important to the trajectory of the longevity meme.

22. I know because I have been been in many meetings with him and glimpsed his calendar during a PowerPoint session.

23. See Gladwell, *The Tipping Point*, 38–58.

24. See http://space.xprize.org/ansari-x-prize.

25. Peter Diamandis, "22nd Century Philanthropy: High Efficiency, High Leverage," Huffington Post, September 3, 2007, www.huffingtonpost.com/peter -diamandis/22nd-century-philanthropy_b_62006.html.

26. Interview with Peter Diamandis, October 11, 2010.

27. Ibid.

28. See http://genomics.xprize.org/.

29. Ibid.

30. Ibid.

31. Ibid.

32. See http://www.mprize.org/.

33. Interview with David Gobel, September 24, 2010.

34. National Cancer Institute, *Cancer Trends Progress Report–2009/2010 Update* (Bethesda, MD: National Cancer Institute, April 2010), http://progress report.cancer.gov.

35. Interview with Gobel.

36. For more information, see www.organovo.com/.

37. Interview with Gobel.

38. See www.foresight.org/about/index.html#Mission.

39. See http://lifeextensionconference.com/. I was a speaker at this conference in October 2010.

40. Nick Bilton, "One on One: Esther Dyson, Health Tech Investor and Space Tourist," *New York Times*, February 26, 2010, http://bits.blogs.nytimes.com/2010/ 02/26/one-on-one-esther-dyson-health-tech-investor-and-space-tourist/.

41. Interview with angel investor Aydin Senkut, July 25, 2010. For more information, see http://www.fortuneconferences.com/brainstormtech/agenda.html.

42. Interview with Aydin Senkut, August 7, 2010. See also http://techonomy .com.

43. Gladwell, *The Tipping Point*, 43.

44. Bruce and Susan Klein were given the title "founding architects" for their role in helping to start Singularity University. See http://singularityu.org/ about/history/.

45. Interview with Bruce Klein, October 5, 2010.

46. Interview with Kevin Perrott, September 28, 2010.

47. Ibid.

48. Ibid.

49. See www.sens.org/sens-foundation/board.

50. Interview with Perrott.

51. Gladwell, *The Tipping Point*, 139.

52. Ibid.

53. Ibid.

54. A more complete genome draft was released in 2003. See also "How Much Did the Human Genome Project Cost U.S. taxpayers?" www.genome .gov/11006943. The Human Genome Project was an international effort, including the United Kingdom, France, Germany, Japan, and China, although the United States contributed the most financial resources. See "Who Participated in the International Human Genome Project Consortium?" www.genome.gov/ 11006943

55. The genome in 2000 was not exactly complete, and researchers are still working to sequence enough genomes to reach a standard definition of complete. See "President Clinton Announces the Completion of the First Survey of the Entire Human Genome, Hails Public and Private Efforts Leading to This Historic Achievement," Human Genome Project Information, June 25, 2000, www.ornl.gov/sci/techresources/Human_Genome/project/clinton1.shtml; and www.ornl.gov/sci/techresources/Human_Genome/project/clinton2.shtml.

56. Ibid.

57. Steven Levy, "Geek Power: Steven Levy Revisits Tech Titans, Hackers, Idealists," *Wired*, April 19, 2010, www.wired.com/magazine/2010/04/ff_hackers/ all/1.

58. Jeff Bezos, "We Are What We Choose," Princeton University address to the Class of 2010 Baccalaureate, May 30, 2010, www.youtube.com/watch?v =vBmavNoChZc.

59. Nicholas Wade, "Researchers Say They Created a Synthetic Cell," *New York Times*, May 20, 2010, www.nytimes.com/2010/05/21/science/21cell.html.

60. J. Craig Venter and Daniel Gibson, "How We Created the First Synthetic Cell," *Wall Street Journal*, May 26, 2010, http://online.wsj.com/article/ SB10001424052748704026204575266460432676840.html.

61. Ibid.

62. See http://groups.google.com/group/diybio/?pli=1.

63. Mike Wilson, *The Difference Between God and Larry Ellison: *God Doesn't Think He's Larry Ellison* (New York: HarperBusiness Paperback, 2003), 266.

64. www.ellisonfoundation.org/adsp.jsp?key=01misstmnt.

65. "Mr. Ellison said that he would have liked to do molecular biology as an alternative career, so Dr. Lederberg invited the software entrepreneur to work

in his lab at Rockefeller in 1994." See www.ellisonfoundation.org/pfbs.jsp ?p=7.

66. Interview with Peter Thiel, November 11, 2010.

67. Nicola Jones, "Education: Ten Weeks to Save the World," *Nature* 467 (September 15, 2010): 266–268, www.nature.com/news/2010/100915/full/ 467266a.html.

68. See Lucinda K. Southworth, Art B. Owen, and Stuart K. Kim, "Effects of Aging on Mouse Transcriptional Networks," NLM Informatics Training Conference 2007, Stanford University, Stanford, California, June 26–27, 2007, www.nlm.nih.gov/ep/trainingconf2007agenda.html#22.

69. Matt C, "23andMe Struts Its Stuff in NYC During Fashion Week," The Spittoon, September 11, 2008, http://spittoon.23andme.com/2008/09/11/23 andme-struts-its-stuff-in-nyc-during-fashion-week/.

70. Andrew Pollack, "Google Co-founder Backs Vast Parkinson's Study," *New York Times*, March 11, 2009, www.nytimes.com/2009/03/12/business/12 gene.html?_r=1.

71. Leena Rao, "While 23andMe Raises $11 Million, Mohr Davidow Sells Stake to Invest in Rival," TechCrunch, May 4, 2009, http://techcrunch.com/ 2009/05/04/while-23andme-raises-11-million-mohr-davidow-sells-stake-to -invest-in-rival/.

72. Thomas Goetz, "Sergey Brin's Search for a Parkinson's Cure," *Wired*, June 22, 2010, www.wired.com/magazine/2010/06/ff_sergeys_search/.

73. Ibid.

74. Interview with Mike Kope, November 11, 2010.

75. Allen Institute, "Paul G. Allen Commits $100 Million to Brain Research," press release, September 16, 2003, www.alleninstitute.org/Media/ documents/press_releases/09_16_03_PressRelease.pdf.

76. Ibid.

77. Allen Institute, "Allen Institute for Brain Science Launches Three New Landmark Atlas Projects Focusing on the Human Brain, Developing Brain and Spinal Cord," press release, March 13, 2008, www.alleninstitute.org/ Media/documents/press_releases/2008_0313_PressRelease_NewProjects.pdf.

78. National Institutes of Health, "NIH Launches the Human Connectome Project to Unravel the Brain's Connections," press release, July 15, 2009, www .nih.gov/news/health/jul2009/ninds-15.htm. See also www.humanconnectome .org/consortia/.

79. See Dharmendra Modha's blog motto, http://modha.org/blog/2008/11/ ibm_awarded_darpa_funding_via_1.html. See also http://bluebrain.epfl.ch/.

80. Natasha Singer, "The Financial Time Bomb of Longer Lives," *New York Times*, October 16, 2010, www.nytimes.com/2010/10/17/business/17stream .html?_r=2.

81. Ibid.

82. Michael J. Rae, Robert N. Butler, Judith Campisi et al., "The Demographic and Biomedical Case for Late-Life Interventions in Aging," *Science Translational Medicine* 2, no. 24 (July 14, 2010): 1.

83. Ibid.

84. Ibid., 2.

85. S. Jay Olshansky, Daniel Perry, Richard A. Miller, and Robert N. Butler, "In Pursuit of the Longevity Dividend: What Should We Be Doing to Prepare for the Unprecedented Aging of Humanity?" *The Scientist*, March 2006, 32.

86. Some may argue that the government spends more than this on anti-aging if one includes work done in areas such as cancer research and Alzheimer's. The above number is the clearest figure for research focused on understanding the mechanisms of aging. As Daniel Perry from the Alliance for Aging Research said in an interview on March 25, 2011, "The exact number for the government's anti-aging budget depends on who you ask and how you define anti-aging." The NIH Almanac–Appropriations, section 2, US Department of Health and Human Services, 2009 figures, http://www.nih.gov/about/almanac/appropriations/part2.htm. Aging Biology Budget, National Institute on Aging, US National Institutes of Health, 2009 actual budget, http://www.nia.nih.gov/NR/exeres/B9D30A3D-8D44-447F-82B2-D5770FF95575.htm.

87. Peter W. Huber, "The FDA and Methuselah," Forbes.com, April 12, 2010, www.manhattan-institute.org/html/miarticle.htm?id=6063.

88. Rae et al., "The Demographic and Biomedical Case," 4.

Index

Acron Cell Company, 186
Adam and Eve, 2–3, 4
Adenovirus, 35
Adoption, 124
Adulthood/adultolescents, 109,
    110–113
AFIRM. *See* Armed Forces Institute
    of Regenerative Medicine
Afterlife, 154, 163, 173
Ageless: The Naked Truth About
    Bioidentical Hormones
    (Somers), 17
Aging, 22–24, 40(fig.), 44, 45, 81,
    105, 167, 175, 178, 183, 196
  age differences in relationships/
    siblings, 113–117, 119
  anti-aging therapies, 197
  and business leaders, 137
  chronological vs. biological age,
    177
  delayed by seven years, 196
  growth of older/younger
    populations, 195
  plasticity of, 37–39, 47, 195, 198
  search for antiaging pill, 39–42
Aging Research Network, 186
Agriculture, 59

AI. *See* Artificial intelligence
AIDS, 37, 96
Airlines, 68
Alchemists, 13
Alcohol consumption, 3–4
Alexander the Great, 12–13
Algae, 67, 68
Alginate hydrogel, 107
Allen, Paul, 138, 181, 190, 193–194
Allen, Woody, 151
Allen Institute for Brain Science
    (Seattle), 193–194
Alm, Richard, 95, 96
Alzheimer's, 22, 39, 194, 197
Ambition, 139–142, 149
American Council on Science and
    Health, 59
American Federation of Labor-
    Congress of Industrial
    Organizations, 74
Ames, Bruce, 185
Anatomy of Love (Fisher), 111
Angola, 92
Annas, George, 90, 91
Antibiotics, 22, 131
Apple Inc., 138
Aquinas, St. Thomas, 5

Archimedes, 139
Archon Genomics X PRIZE, 181, 182
Aristotle, 162
Armed Forces Institute of Regenerative Medicine (AFIRM), 30
Arnett, Dr. Jeffrey Jensen, 111
Art, 171
Artemisinin, 67
Arteriocyte company, 31
Artificial intelligence (AI), 179, 180, 181, 191
Artificial life, 188, 189
Asian American females, 92
Asimov, Isaac, 10
Association of Medical Practitioners and Dentists (Italy), 102
Astrology, 15–16
Atala, Dr. Anthony, 26–27, 28, 30
AT&T, 58
Atheists/agnostics, 155(fig.), 158, 159, 160, 161, 163, 164
Atwood, Joan D., 124
Australia, 82–83, 124, 136
Authoritarianism, 85
AutoFarm, 50

Bacon, Francis, 14–15
Bacon, Roger, 2, 15
Badylak, Dr. Stephen, 28–29, 30
Bailey, Ronald, 85
Bangladesh, 54
Banks, 146
Barzilai, Dr. Nir, 44
Bathory, Elizabeth, 8–9
Becker, Ernest, 151
Becker, Gary, 128–129, 132–133
Belief systems and College Graduates, 159 (table), 161(table)
Belkin, Lisa, 101
Bequests, 146

Berger, Peter, 153, 154, 156
Bergholdt, Stinne Holm, 105
Bezos, Jeff, 188–189
Bhatia, Dr. Mick, 32, 33
Bible, 2–3, 164
Bicentennial Man, The (Asimov), 10
Bill and Melinda Gates Foundation, 67, 80. *See also* Gates, Bill
Biofuels, 67, 68
Biogerontology, 183
Bioidentical hormone replacement therapy, 17, 18
Biology, 190–194
  bioinformatics, 188, 198
  do-it-yourself biology (DIY), 189–190
  as engineering project, 46 (*see also* Human Genome Project; Tissue engineering)
  as information technology, 44
  new/smart biology, 185
  synthetic biology, 45, 67, 189
Biotech Humanitarian Award, 67
Biotechnology, access to, 92–93, 94, 95, 96
"Birthmark, The" (Hawthorne), 77
Birth rate, 119. *See also* Fertility rates
Blackburn, Dr. Elizabeth, 41
Bladders, 26–27
Blade Runner (film), 1
Blair, Tony, 188
Blasco, Dr. Maria, 38
Blindness, 33, 35, 36(fig.)
Blood pharming, 31
Blood pressure, 44
Blood transfusions, 14
Blood vessels, 28
Bloom, David, 130
Blue Brain Project, 194
Blumwald, Dr. Eduardo, 59
Boia, Lucian, 3, 7
Bone marrow treatment, 37

Boomers, 146, 149, 195
Borlaug, Norman, 59
Boston University New England
    Centenarian Study, 44
Bostrom, Nick, 88
Boudreaux, Donald, 139
Bousada, Carmen, 102
Braga, David, 50
Brains, 163, 179, 188, 193–194
    mapping human brain, 194
Brazil, 157
Brin, Sergey, 138, 190, 192–193
Brown, Louise, 103
Brown, Timothy, 37
Brown-Séquard, Charles-Edouard, 5
Bubble boy disease, 35–36, 83
Buck Institute, 186
Burn repair, 30, 33
Burson, Harold, 137
Bush, George W., 78, 80
BusinessWeek magazine, 137, 138
Butler, Dr. Robert, 195

Caenorhabditis elegans, 38
Callahan, Daniel, 80–81
Calment, Jeanne, 2
Caloric restriction (CR), 17, 39,
    40(fig.), 176, 177, 195–196
Calories, intake per capita, 55,
    55(fig.)
Cameron, Nigel M. de S., 166
Cancer, 22, 23, 29, 36–37, 38–39,
    42, 44, 73, 79, 84, 102, 104,
    105, 107, 196, 197
    cost of cancer care, 183
Cane toads, 82–83
Canning, David, 130
Capital accumulation, 143
Caplan, Arthur, 79
Carbon emissions, 63, 67, 68
Cardiovascular disease, 44. *See also*
    Hearts: heart disease

Careers, multiple, 139–140, 149,
    166, 167
Carnes, Bruce A., 5, 14
Carr, Elizabeth Jordan, 103
Carter, Jimmy, 80
Casscells, Dr. S. Ward, 30
Castillo, Claudia, 24–25
Catholics, 154, 160, 162, 165
CDC. *See* Centers for Disease
    Control and Prevention
Celebrity culture, 169
Celera Genomics, 4, 187
Cell, 39
Cell phones, 63, 95
Cellular/molecular damage, 46(fig.)
Centenarians, 44, 144
Centeno-Schultz Clinic (Broomfield,
    Colorado), 34
Center for Responsible
    Nanotechnology (CRN), 74
Center for Retirement Research at
    Boston College, 146
Center for Third Age
    Leadership, 112
Centers for Disease Control and
    Prevention (CDC), 106, 121
Central Intelligence Agency, 92
Chaplin, Charlie, 101
Chapman, Dr. Audrey, 87, 88
Chemotherapy, 104, 105
Childbearing, 105–106, 107(fig.),
    112, 122–123, 158
Childlessness, 119–121
Children's Hospital of
    Philadelphia, 35
China, 157
Christensen, Clayton, 135
Chronic Fatigue Syndrome, 179
Church, Dr. George, 186
Cinnabar, 13
Civil rights, 64, 65(fig.)
Clement, James, 186

Clinton, Bill, 43, 64, 80, 176, 179, 188
Coady, C. A. J., 82–83
Coal, 70, 72
Cocoon (film), 11
Cohabitation, 110
Cold fusion, 68–69
Cole-Turner, Ronald, 152–153
Collins, Dr. Francis, 42, 44, 160
Colorado Center for Reproductive Medicine (CCRM), 104–105
Complete Genomics, 43
Compound interest, 147, 150
ComputerLand Corporation, 186
Computers, 95, 136, 171, 179, 185. *See also* Internet
Concordia University (Canada), 116
Conferences, 184, 185
Connectors, 181–186
Conservation, 64
Contraception, 119
Copper, 58
Cordell, Joe, 177
Council of the Indies, 13
Coursey, Don, 60–61
Cox, Michael, 95, 96
CR. *See* Caloric restriction
Creation Museum in Kentucky, 156
Creativity, 1, 2, 11, 57, 58, 80, 135, 138, 140
Crichton, Michael, 71
Crizotinib, 83–84
Cro-Magnon era, 21
Cryonics, 18–19, 171
Cutter Laboratories, 83
Cytokines, 32

Daoists, 167. *See also* Taoism
DARPA. *See* Defense Advanced Research Projects Agency
da Vinci, Leonardo, 140
Dawkins, Richard, 158

Death, 79, 81, 82, 89, 102, 115, 123, 149, 151, 172, 190, 194, 197
  child mortality rates, 119
  death rates, 52–53, 54, 119
  as fault of humans, 2–6, 19
  overcoming/fighting, 6–20, 152, 167, 170, 191
  and sex, 6
  undead (term), 7
  See also under Religion
DeBaets, Amy Michelle, 166
Debt, 195
Deepwater Horizon oil spill, 70
Defense Advanced Research Projects Agency (DARPA), 31, 45, 194
Deforestation, 62
de Grey, Dr. Aubrey, 45, 120, 178–179, 183, 184, 191
Democracy, 64, 65(fig.)
Denis, Jean, 15
Developing countries, 91–92, 131–132, 134
Devi, Rajo, 101, 102
Diabetes, 37, 39, 41
Diamandis, Peter, 181–182, 185
Dictators, 89
Diet, 3, 15, 16–17
  books about diet and longevity, 16
  See also Caloric restriction; Nutrition
Difference, The (Page), 96
Discover magazine, 67
Diseases, 22, 24, 33, 35–36, 43, 47, 78, 79, 81, 83, 95, 131, 179, 188, 190, 192–193, 194, 195, 196–197
Disrupting Class (Christensen), 136
Divorce, 111, 114, 124, 167
DNA, 31, 37, 67, 95, 97, 189, 192
  DNA synthesis, 188
  mitochondrial, 179
  See also Genes/gene therapy; Human Genome Project

Donley, Carol C., 9
Dorff, Rabbi Elliot N., 152, 166
Doust-Blazy, Dr. Philippe, 102
D'Souza, Dinesh, 164
Dublin, Louis, 23
DuPont, 73, 74
Dworkin, Ronald, 86
Dyson, Ester, 184, 185

ECM. *See* Extracellular matrix
Economic growth, 61, 64, 97, 98, 128, 129, 131, 134, 135, 140, 148
Economic life of individuals, 127–128
Economist, The, 64, 66, 152, 153, 156
Education, 53, 92, 98, 111, 112, 118, 122, 132–137, 143, 149, 167
    and religion, 157–163
    and unemployment/earnings, 134(fig.)
"Effects of Aging on Mouse Transcriptional Networks" (Southworth and Kim), 192
Egypt, 132
Ehrlich, Paul, 54, 56, 58
EKC. *See* Environmental Kuznets curve
Electricity, 95, 140
Eliade, Mircea, 16
Elixirs, 13–14
Ellison, Larry, 190
Ellison Foundation, 190–191
Elman, Cheryl, 123
El Salvador, 132
Emmett, Ross B., 55
Ending Aging: The Rejuvenation Breakthroughs That Could Reverse Human Aging in Our Lifetime (de Grey), 45
Endocrine system, 17
England, 10, 14, 56, 65, 66, 103
Entrepreneurs, 97, 98
Environmental Defense Fund, 73, 74

Environmental issues, 60–66, 75
    oil spills, 70
    and wealth, 63
    See also Global warming; Pollution
Environmental Kuznets curve (EKC), 61–62, 62(fig.)
Enzymes, 37, 39, 45
Eos and Tithonus, 10
Epic of Gilgamesh, The, 5–6
Episcopal church, 165
Esophageal cancer, 29
Essay on the Principle of Population (Malthus), 54
ETC group, 72
Ettinger, Robert, 19
Eugenics, 84, 85, 94
Evolution, 157–158, 160, 168
Extracellular matrix (ECM), 24, 29, 30
ExxonMobil, 68

Facebook, 191
Facial reconstruction, 30
Faith, 172
Family, 101–125, 147
    extended/mixed families, 123–125
    shared stories/memories in, 117–118
    size and structure, 119–123, 120(table)
Famines, 54
Fantastic Voyage: How to Live Long Enough to Live Forever (Kurzweil and Grossman), 180
Fashion Week (New York), 192
Faust theme, 6–8
FDA. *See* Food and Drug Administration
Fertility rates, 52, 53, 54, 119, 121, 122(fig.), 123
Fertility technology/clinics, 102–108, 114

Fiber optics, 58
Fisher, Dr. Helen, 111
Fisher, Irving, 144
Five Minds for the Future
     (Gardner), 135
Fleischmann, Martin, 68–69
Fohr, Sherry E., 152, 166
Foltz, Dr. Greg, 194
Food and Drug Administration
     (FDA), 17, 31, 33, 34, 196–197
Food shortages, 50
Foresight Institute, 71–71, 184
Fortune Tech Brainstorm (2010), 185
Founder's Fund, 191
Fountain of youth, 11, 12
Frankenstein monster, 8, 19, 71, 82
Franklin, Benjamin, 17, 140
Freitas, Robert, 180
French paradox, 3
Freud, Sigmund, 162
Fukuyama, Francis, 89–90, 91, 92, 94
Funding, 183, 194, 195, 196
Furstenberg, Frank F., 111

Garden of Eden, 2–3. *See also*
     Adam and Eve
Gardner, Howard, 135
Gates, Bill, 54, 57, 67, 80, 138, 170,
     180, 188, 189
Gavrilov, Dr. Leonid, 52
Gavrilova, Dr. Natalia, 52
Gays, 165
GDP. *See* Gross domestic product
Gehry, Frank, 192
Gelsinger, Jesse, 83
Generation issues, 166
     Generation Y, 135–136, 149
     growth of older/younger
          populations, 195
Genes/gene therapy, 31, 34–37,
     38–39, 47, 67, 83–84, 95, 179,
     191, 194

genetic engineering, 90
synthetic genome, 189
transgenes, 35
VMAT2 gene, 163
Genetic warfare, 91
Geniuses, 57
Genocide, 90
Geron company, 33, 41
Gibson, Daniel, 189
Gilgamesh, 5
Gladwell, Malcolm, 176, 185, 187
GlaxoSmithKline, 40, 191
Global economy, 135
Global positioning system (GPS),
     49–50
Global warming, 64, 68
Globe and Mail (Canada), 58
Goals, 143, 146
Gobel, David, 183–184
God, 2, 99, 153, 159, 162, 168, 171
     playing God, 83, 86
     See also Religion
Godbey, Dr. Geoffrey, 128, 142
God Gene, The (Hamer), 163
God Is Back (Micklethwait and
          Wooldridge), 157
Goertzel, Dr. Ben, 179
Goethe, Johann Wolfgang von, 7
Goetz, Thomas, 193
Gold, 13
Golombok, Susan, 125
Gonadotropin cycle, 103
Goodman, Ellen, 77
Goodness, 172
Google, 63, 138
Gordon, Linda Perlman, 111
Gounod, Charles, 7
GPS. *See* Global positioning system
GQ magazine, 178–179
Grafts of animal/human tissue, 17, 33
Greek mythology, 4, 10–11
Greeley, Andrew M., 154–156

Green, Jarvis, 34
Greenpeace, 74
Grim, Dr. Brian, 156
Gross domestic product (GDP), 119,
    120(table), 131
Grossman, Gene, 61, 62
Grossman, Dr. Terry, 180
Group identity/interests, 116–117, 163
Gruman, Gerald, 4, 13
Guggenheim, Davis, 135
Gulliver's Travels (Swift), 9–10, 19
Gupta, Dr. Sanjay, 175–176, 178

Haas, Corey, 35, 84
Habits, 3
Hackler, Chris, 140–141
Haiti, 80
Halcyon Molecular, 191
Hamer, Dean, 163
Hari, Johann, 84–85
Harried Leisure Class, The
    (Linder), 129
Harris, John, 81, 82
Hawking, Stephen, 182
Hawthorne, Nathaniel, 77
Haycock, David Boyd, 3, 10
"Health and Wealth of Nations, The"
    (Bloom and Canning), 130
Health care, 146, 147, 156, 183,
    185, 195
Health span, 45, 47, 51, 63, 66, 108,
    115, 135, 136, 137, 139, 140,
    158, 170, 177, 195, 198. *See also*
    Wealth: and health
Hearts, 148
    growing rat/pig hearts in lab, 27
    heart disease, 4, 22, 23, 27, 33, 39,
        44, 182, 196, 197
    heart valves, 177
Helping others, 86–87
Henry VI, 14
Hernandez, Isaias (Corporal), 30

Hessel, Andrew, 95
Heylin, John, 172
HGH. *See* Human growth hormone
HGP. *See* Human Genome Project
Hierarchy of needs, 60, 61(fig.), 62
Higgins, Dr. E. Tory, 118
High, Dr. Katherine A., 35
Hill, Peter, 168–169
Hines, Jean, 143
HIV, 37
Hobbes, Thomas, 78
Holliday, Chad, 73
Homebrew Club, 190
Hood, Ralph, 168–169
Hook, C. Christopher, 84
Hormones, 17–18, 38
Housing, 156
Hout, Michael, 154–156
Howard, Ron, 11
Huber, Peter, 60, 196
Hughes, James, 94
Human capital, 128, 130, 132, 134,
    138, 142, 143
Human Connectome Project, 194
Human development index, 122(fig.)
Human Genome Project (HGP),
    42–44, 95, 181–182, 187
Human growth hormone (HGH),
    17–18
Human nature, 79, 80, 89–90, 115
Human rights, 90
Hurlbut, William, 83
Hybrid cars, 63

IAC/InterActive Corporation, 192
Iannaccone, Lawrence, 153, 157,
    167–168
IBM, 60, 194
Ideas, 57–58, 97, 98, 187
Immortality, 3, 8–13, 52, 80, 151,
    152–153
    as a curse, 7, 10

Immortality Institute, 186
Income, 60–61, 62–63, 65, 92, 130.
    See also Wages; Wealth
India, 59, 65–66, 101, 157
Industrial revolution, 73
Inflammation, 35, 44
Information technology, 44, 95
Information vs. knowledge, 171
Infrastructure, 58
Inglehart, Ronald, 154, 156, 162
Inheritance, 146, 147
Innovation, 57–58, 98, 197
"In Pursuit of the Longevity
    Dividend" (Olshansky, Perry
    et al.), 196
Institute of Biotechnology and the
    Human Future, 84
Insulin resistance, 44
Insurance, 86, 87
Intel, 60
Internet, 95, 99, 120, 142, 146, 149,
    156, 157, 177, 186, 193
    Internet Corporation for Assigned
    Names and Numbers, 184–185
Inventions, 140. *See also* Innovation
Investments, 147, 191
In vitro fertilization (IVF), 103,
    104, 105
Islam, 166–167
Italy, 102
IVF. *See* In vitro fertilization

Jain religion, 152, 165–166
"Jameson Satellite, The" (Jones), 18
Jenkins, Mark Collins, 8, 9
Jews, 154, 166
Job market, 138, 149. *See also* Labor
    force; Work
Jobs, Steve, 138, 190
John Deere tractors, 49–50
Johnson, Dr. Todd, 154, 156
Joint repair, 34

Jones, Dr. Howard and
    Dr. Georgeanna, 102–103
Jones, Neil Ronald, 18
Journaling, 169
Journal of Neuroscience, 32
Joy, Bill, 71
June, Dr. Carl, 37

Kamm, Frances, 87
Kant, Immanuel, 87
Kaplan, Jordan, 135–136
Karma, 165, 166
Kass, Dr. Leon, 77, 78–79, 81
Keasling, Dr. Jay, 67
Kefalas, Maria, 109
Keirstead, Dr. Hans, 32–33
Keller, Bill, 169
Kennedy, John F., 118
Kent, Dr. Craig, 28
Kenyon, Dr. Cynthia, 38, 191
Kim, Dr. Stuart K., 192
King, Larry, 182
Klaus, Frank, 17
Klein, Bruce, 185–186
Klug, Aaron, 37
Knowledge, 171, 172
Kohn, Livia, 167
Kope, Mike, 193
Kotelko, Olga, 23
Kristof, Nicholas D., 162–163
Krueger, Alan, 61, 62
Krupp, Fred, 73
Kula, Witold, 124
Kulkarni, Deepa, 29
Kurzweil, Ray, 69, 74, 95–96,
    170–172, 179–180, 185

Labor Department, 108
Labor force, 108–109, 119, 137, 138,
    140–141, 143. *See also* Work
Lactic acid, 16
Laderman, Gary, 168–169, 169–170

Lamarckism, 5
LaMonica, Martin, 60
Landfills, 65–66
Lane, Robert W., 50–51
Law of Accelerating Returns, 70, 96
LCA. *See* Leber congenital amaurosis
Leachate, 65–66
Leadership, 165
Leber congenital amaurosis (LCA),
    35, 84
Lederberg, Dr. Joshua, 191
Leisure, 132, 142–142, 143, 148
Leukemia, 83
Liberty University, 157
Life cycle hypothesis, 145
Life expectancy, 17, 46, 47, 51,
    65, 88, 98, 99, 102, 104, 109,
    110, 112, 129
  countries ranked for, 93(table)
  disparities in, 91–92, 94
  growth for men and women, 137
  and number of evenings/weekends,
    141(fig.)
  objections to extending, 77–78,
    78–89
  of 150 years, 47, 52, 81, 107, 113,
    140, 141, 143, 145, 177, 180
  over time, 21, 22(fig.), 23
  and wealth, 131
Life span, 2–3, 17, 51, 128
  and concern for the
    environment, 63
  of mice, 39
  of worms, 38
  See also Health span; Life
    expectancy; Longevity
LifeStar Institute, 186
Limb ischemia, 33
Linder, Staffan, 129
Literature, 171
Logan, Barbara, 186
London, Andrew, 123

Longevity, 12–20, 53, 77–99, 114,
    115, 122, 123, 130–131, 176
  countries' share of welfare
    improvements due to gains in,
    133(fig.)
  enhancements concerning,
    84–99
  financial implications of, 127–150
  longevity meme, 176, 178–181,
    182, 187, 188, 190, 191, 195
  See also Life expectancy; Life span
Longevity Genes Project (Albert
    Einstein College of Medicine), 44
Lou Gehrig's disease, 33, 182
Lower, Richard, 14
Lugo, Luis E., 161
Lungs, 24–25, 27, 73, 84
Lysosomes, 45

McArthur Foundation Network on
    Transitions to Adulthood, 109
McClintick, David, 56
McGowan Institute for Regenerative
    Medicine, 28
McKibben, Bill, 71, 79
McKubre, Dr., Michael, 69
McMaster University (Ontario),
    31, 32
Macular degeneration, 33, 43–44
Maher, Derek, 152
Malaria, 67, 80
Male fertility, 108
Malthus, Thomas, 54
Manuelli, Rodolfo, 134
Mao Zedong, 163
Markel, Howard, 83
Marriage, 108–110, 112, 158, 162,
    166, 167
  remarriage, 123, 124
Masalla, Luke, 26–27
Maslow, Abraham, 60, 61(fig.),
    62, 162

Mavens, 178–181, 184, 193
Maynard, Andrew, 73
Meaning of life, 162, 172
Media, 113, 146
Medicare, 196
Memes, 175, 187. *See also* Longevity:
    longevity meme
Menopause, 105
Mensa International, 57
Mercer, Calvin, 152, 170
Mercury (metal), 14
Mesothelioma, 73
Metals, 13, 56, 58
Metchnikoff, Elie, 16
Methane, 66
Methuselah, 2
Methuselah Foundation, 191
Mexico, 98, 131
Micklethwait, John, 156–157
Microsoft, 63, 138
Miller, Henry, 59
Mind over matter, 4
Mint (personal finance tool), 146
Mitchell, C. Ben, 84
*Mitochondrial Free Radical Theory of
    Aging, The* (de Grey), 178
MIT Technology Review, 45
Modernity, 153, 154, 156
Modha, Dharmendra, 194
Monaco, 92
Mona Lisa, 140
Monsters, 8. *See also* Frankenstein
    monster
Moore's law, 95, 188
Morality, 3, 7, 81, 82, 87, 102
More, Max, 99
Morris, Bob, 147
Moses, 2
Mprize, 183, 186
Murdoch, Rupert, 101
Murdock, David, 176
Murphy, Keith, 28

Murphy, Kevin, 131
Muscle replacement/growth, 30,
    37, 177
Music, 169, 171
Myrskylä, Dr. Mikko, 121
Myths of Rich and Poor (Alm and
    Cox), 95

Naam, Ramez, 83, 85
Nano Risk Framework, 73
Nanosolar company, 70
Nanotechnology, 68, 69–73, 181, 184
National Academy of Sciences, 57
National Bureau of Economic
    Research, 131
National Cancer Institute, 36–37, 183
National Institute on Aging, 41
National Institutes of Health (NIH),
    42, 194, 196
National Medal of Technology, 179
National Science Foundation, 134
Native Americans, 92
"Natural" labels, 78
Nature, 41
Nazis, 84, 89
New biology, 185
New England Journal of Medicine, 33
Newsweek, 26, 111
New York Times, 8, 16, 23, 41,
    101, 195
Nietzsche, Friedrich, 153
NIH. *See* National Institutes of
    Health
Niklason, Dr. Laura, 27
Noah, 2
Nobel Prize, 16, 59, 61, 139, 191
Nontraded goods, 132
Nonviolence, 165
Norris, Pippa, 154, 156, 162
Novariant company, 50
Nucleases, 37
Nutrition, 22. *See also* Diet

Obama, Barack, 63
Obesity, 55
O'Connor, Michael, 49–50
OECD. *See* Organization for
    Economic Co-operation and
    Development
Oeppen, Jim, 23
Olshansky, S. Jay, 5, 14, 131, 196
Opiates, 13
Oprah Winfrey Show, The, 29
Organization for Economic
    Co-operation and Development
    (OECD), 106, 113, 119, 144
Organ mold, 187
Organovo company, 28, 184
Organ printing, 28, 184
Organ transplants, 15, 105. *See also*
    Regeneration/replacement of
    body parts
Orphans, 124
Ovarian transplant/tissue, 105, 106
Overall, Christine, 94
Oz, Dr. Mehmet, 176–177, 187

Page, Larry, 138, 192
Page, Scott E., 96
Pakistan, 59
Pandora, 3
Paracelsus, 13
Parenting, 112, 115, 118
Parkinson's disease, 179, 192–193
Parvez, Ghulam Ahmed, 166–167
Patience, 137–138
Patterns/patternists, 171, 172
Pedophilia, 162
Perls, Dr. Thomas, 44, 144
Perrott, Kevin, 186
Perry, Daniel, 196
"Personalized Life Extension
    Conference: Anti-Aging
    Strategies for a Long Healthy
    Life" (conference), 184

Personalized medicine, 192
Peterson, Christine, 72, 184, 185
Peterson, Dr. Michael, 29
Pew Forum on Religious and Public
    Life, 159
Pew Research Center, 160
    Social and Demographic Trends
    survey on aging, 23
Phoenix, Chris, 74
Picture of Dorian Gray, The (Wilde), 6
Pink Army Cooperative, 95
Pinochet, Augusto, 89
Placebo effect, 5, 17
Plec, Julie, 8
Pluralism, religious, 156
Political issues, 84, 85, 89, 91
Pollution, 50, 51, 60, 63, 68, 78
Ponce de León, Juan, 12
Pons, Stanley, 68–69
Popenoe, David, 110
Population Bomb, The (Ehrlich), 54
Population growth, 50, 51, 52–53,
    53(fig.), 59, 75
    and innovative ideas, 57–58
*Population Growth and Economic
    Development* (National Academy
    of Sciences), 57
Posner, Richard, 140
Poverty, 87, 88, 94, 97, 130, 156
Precautionary principle, 74
President's Council on Bioethics,
    77, 78
Preston, Samuel, 57
Prey (Crichton), 71
Prices, 55, 56–57, 58–59, 70, 95, 97
Productivity, 130, 140, 141–142, 148
Prometheus, 4
Property and Environment Research
    Center, 56
Property rights, 64, 65(fig.)
Prospect of Immortality, The
    (Ettinger), 19

Qin Shi Huang, 14
Quality of life, 21, 34
Quest for Immortality, The
    (Olshansky and Carnes), 5, 14
Question of Blood, A (Rankin), 117

Race, 94
Rankin, Ian, 117
Rapamycin, 41
Raskin, Virginia, 127
Rational choice theory, 167
Rational Optimist, The (Ridley), 97
Rats, 27, 32–33
Raw materials, 56
RealAge.com, 177
Recker, Nancy, 115
Recycling, 65
Redstone, Sumner, 137
Refrigeration, 15, 78
Regeneration/replacement of body
    parts, 13, 24–25, 25(fig.), 26,
    29–31, 177, 187
Regenerative medicine, 30, 32. *See
    also* Regeneration/replacement
    of body parts
Regenerus, Mark, 109
Regenexx procedure, 34
Rejuvenation, 12, 13, 14, 15, 183
Rejuvenation Research (journal),
    42, 52
Religion, 1–2, 151–173
    college graduates and belief
        systems, 159(table), 161(table)
    and death, 162
    fundamentalists, 158, 160, 168
    percent of population
        belonging to religion or no
        religion, 155(fig.)
    unexpected religious movements,
        169
    See also Bible, God; *under*
        Education

*Religion and the Implications of Radical
    Life Extension* (Maher, Mercer,
    and Dorff), 152
Renaissance era, 21
Renouncers, 165–166
Reproductive technology, 101,
    123, 125. *See also* Fertility
    technology/clinics
Resource depletion/allocation, 57, 87.
    See also Food shortages
Resveratrol, 39, 40, 41, 191
Retirement, 140, 143–144,
    145, 149
Reverse engineering, 194
Ridley, Matt, 97–98
Rituals, 169, 170, 171, 172
Robinson, Dr. John P., 128, 142
Robots/robotics, 70, 71, 181
Roizen, Dr. Michael, 177
Romer, Paul, 97, 98
Röntgen, Wilhelm Conrad, 140
Roosevelt, Franklin D., 143
Rose, Charlie, 71
Rosenberg, Dr. Steven, 36–37
Rumbaut, Rubén G. 111
Rutan, Burt, 181

Sacredness, 168–169
Sadler, Dr. William, 112
Safety issues, 73–74, 78, 83
Safina, Carl, 64
Sagan, Carl, 153
Salamanders, 13, 28
Saletan, William, 101
Salinity, 59
Sandel, Michael, 86
Sangamo BioSciences, 37
Sanitation, 22, 51
Savings, 144–148, 149
Scarless wound healing, 30
Schmookler Reis, Dr. Robert J., 38
Schönpflug, Ute, 118

Science, 1, 19, 21, 69, 77, 101,
    107, 151, 152, 153, 169, 170,
    171, 172
  science-based education, 158
  scientists' belief in God, 160
Scientist, 196
Secularism, 153, 154, 156, 157
Self-actualization, 148
Self-awareness, 112, 169
Self-replicating machines, 71
Self-transcendence, 163
SENS. *See* Strategies for Engineered
    Negligible Senescence
Seshadri, Ananth, 134
Settersten, Richard A., 111
Severe combined immunodeficiency,
    36
Sex, 5, 110, 114
Shaffer, Susan Morris, 111
Shared memories, 117, 118
Shaw, George Bernard, 4–5
Shelley, Mary, 8
Shepherd Center (Atlanta), 33
Sherkat, Darren, 158–159
Siblings, 115–116, 118, 119
Simon, Julian, 56, 57,
    129–130
Sinclair, David, 39, 40, 41, 191
Singularity Institute for Artificial
    Intelligence, 191
Singularity Is Near, The (Kurzweil),
    170–171, 180
Singularity movement, 170–172
Singularity University (SU),
    180–181, 185, 186, 191, 192
Sirtris Pharmaceuticals, 40–41, 191
Sirtuins, 39, 40
60 Minutes, 29, 69, 152
Skin cancer, 36–37
Skin cells, 31–32, 33
Small, Meredith, 114
Small businesses, 138

Smart biology, 185
Smithsonian Museum of Natural
    History, 157
Snakes, 5, 14
Social change, 186
Social epidemics, 187
Social justice, 88, 89, 94
Social Network, The (film), 191
Social security, 143, 156
Solar power, 68, 69–70
Somers, Suzanne, 18
South Korea, 98
Southworth, Lucy, 192
Spain's National Cancer Research
    Center, 38
Sperm cells, 108, 125
Spilka, Bernard, 168–169
Spinal injuries, 32
Spirituality, 161, 163, 168, 169, 172.
    See also Religion
Spit parties, 192
Sports, 140, 142
Sprint, 63
Sprott, Richard, 190–191
Stallone, Sylvester, 17
Standard and Poor's, 195
Standard of living, 57, 97, 145
Stargardt's macular dystrophy, 33
Statistics Norway, 113
Stem cells, 24, 26, 31, 32–34, 47, 77,
    108. *See also* Skin cells
Stern, Alexandra Minna, 83
Stevenson, Betsey, 111
Stickiness factor, 186–187
Stipp, David, 39
Stockholm syndrome, 88
Stoker, Bram, 7
Stoning children who disobey, 164
Strategies for Engineered Negligible
    Senescence (SENS), 45,
    46(fig.), 178, 191
Substance abuse, 159, 169

Suspended animation, 18
Suzuki, Osamu, 137
Sweden, 52, 53
Swift, Jonathan, 9–10, 19
Swing, Bishop William E., 164–165
Synthetic biology, 45, 67, 189
Synthetic Genomics, 67

Taoism, 4, 167
TA Sciences, 41
TA-65 telomerase activator, 41
Taylor, Dr. Doris, 27
T cells, 37
Technology, 21, 87, 95, 98, 99, 132,
    138, 141–142, 149, 151, 169,
    170, 171, 195. *See also*
    Biotechnology, access to;
    Information technologies;
    Reproductive technology
Techonomy conference in Tahoe, 185
TED conference, 178
Telomerase, 38, 41–42
Telomeres, 41–42
Terrorist attacks of September 11,
    2001, 118, 156
Terry, Lara, 144
Test-tube babies, 103
Thailand, 54
"Theory of the Allocation
    of Time, A" (Becker), 128
Thiel, Peter, 185, 190, 191, 198
Time concept, 1, 109, 148–150, 198
    economic value of time, 128–129
Time magazine, 28
Tipping Point, The (Gladwell), 176
Tissue engineering, 26, 47, 148
Tobacco, 13, 14
Topel, Robert, 131
Trachea, 24, 25(fig.)
Training, 136, 141, 143
Transcendence, 163, 171, 172
Transhumanism, 170

Transistors, 95
Trauma repair, 30
Treder, Mike, 74
True Blood (HBO series), 8
Truth, 161, 164–165, 169
Tuberculosis, 24
Turkey, 157
Turtles, 182
23andMe company, 95, 97, 184, 192
Twilight movie series, 8

Uncertainty, 145
United Nations, 23, 52, 53, 54
United Religious Initiative (URI), 165
United States, life expectancy in, 92
Urban Tribes (Watters), 112, 114
URI. *See* United Religious Initiative
U.S. Bureau of Labor Statistics, 142
U.S. Department of Energy, 42, 67
U.S. National Long-Term Care
    Survey, 23–24

Vaccines, 22, 78, 79, 83, 99, 189
Values, 118–119, 169
Vampires, 7, 19
Vandre, Dr. Robert, 31
Vaupel, James, 23
Venezuela, 132
Venter, Dr. Craig, 44, 67–68, 95, 182,
    187, 189–190
Venture capitalists, 184, 185, 191
Veolia Environment Group, 66
Virtual reality, 136–137, 149
Viruses, 35
Vitamins, 22, 171
Vitrification process, 19, 104–105
Voronoff, Serge, 16
Vouchers, 85

Wages, 135, 143. *See also* Income
Waiting for Superman (documentary),
    135

Wake Forest Institute for
  Regenerative Medicine, 26
Wall Street Journal, 73, 189
Wal-Mart, 63
Warneryd, Karl-Erik, 145
Waste management, 60, 64–67
Water issues, 59, 60, 65–66, 70, 78
Watson, James, 43
Watters, Ethan, 112, 114
Wealth, 53, 54, 60, 62, 61, 73, 87,
  92, 94, 96, 119, 121, 122, 123,
  128, 140, 142, 148, 162
  and health, 129–132
  and religion, 156
  See also Income; *under* Life
  expectancy
Weiner, Jonathan, 89
Welch, Jack, 149
Western Europe, 157
Wheat, 55, 59
Whitaker, Tobias, 4
Wilde, Oscar, 6
Willpower, 5, 6
Wilson, Edward O., 163
Wilson, Mike, 190
Wine, 3–4

Winfrey, Oprah, 169, 176, 187
Wired News/Wired Magazine, 45, 56,
  71, 188
Wojcicki, Anne, 192
Wolf, Dr. Steven, 30
Women, 158. *See also* Childbearing;
  Childlessness; Marriage
Woodruff, Dr. Teresa, 107
Wooldridge, Adrian, 157
Work, 142–144. *See also* Labor force
World Bank, 23, 52
World Summit on Sustainable
  Development, 72
Worms, 38
Wozniak, Steve, 138, 190

X-Men films, 90
X PRIZE, 181

Yeast cells, 67
Yeats, William Butler, 16
Yoga, 15
Young people, 129–130, 138, 149, 195

Zeus, 10
Zinc finger nucleases, 37